Emerging Imaging Technologies in Dentomaxillofacial Radiology

Editors

RUJUTA A. KATKAR
HASSEM GEHA

DENTAL CLINICS OF NORTH AMERICA

www.dental.theclinics.com

July 2018 • Volume 62 • Number 3

ELSEVIER

1600 John F. Kennedy Boulevard • Suite 1800 • Philadelphia, Pennsylvania, 19103-2899

http://www.dental.theclinics.com

DENTAL CLINICS OF NORTH AMERICA Volume 62, Number 3
July 2018 ISSN 0011-8532, ISBN: 978-0-323-61076-6

Editor: John Vassallo; j.vassallo@elsevier.com
Developmental Editor: Laura Fisher

Dental Clinics of North America (ISSN 0011-8532) is published quarterly by Elsevier Inc., 360 Park Avenue South, New York, NY 10010-1710. Months of issue are January, April, July, and October. Business and Editorial Offices: 1600 John F. Kennedy Boulevard, Suite 1800, Philadelphia, PA 19103-2899. Periodicals postage paid at New York, NY and additional mailing offices. Subscription prices are $294.00 per year (domestic individuals), $581.00 per year (domestic institutions), $100.00 per year (domestic students/residents), $364.00 per year (Canadian individuals), $751.00 per year (Canadian institutions), $422.00 per year (international individuals), $751.00 per year (international institutions), and $200.00 per year (international and Canadian students/residents). International air speed delivery is included in all *Clinics* subscription prices. All prices are subject to change without notice. **POSTMASTER:** Send address changes to *Dental Clinics of North America*, Elsevier Health Sciences Division, Subscription Customer Service, 3251 Riverport Lane, Maryland Heights, MO 63043. **Customer Service (orders, claims, online, change of address): Elsevier Health Sciences Division, Subscription Customer Service, 3251 Riverport Lane, Maryland Heights, MO 63043. Tel: 1-800-654-2452 (U.S. and Canada). Fax: 314-447-8029. E-mail: journalscustomer service-usa@elsevier.com (for print support); journalsonlinesupport-usa@elsevier.com (for online support).**

Reprints. For copies of 100 or more, of articles in this publication, please contact the Commercial Reprints Department, Elsevier Inc., 360 Park Avenue South, New York, NY 10010-1710. Tel.: 212-633-3874; Fax: 212-633-3820; E-mail: reprints@elsevier.com.

The *Dental Clinics of North America* is covered in *MEDLINE/PubMed (Index Medicus)*, *Current Contents/Clinical Medicine*, *ISI/BIOMED* and *Clinahl*.

Contributors

EDITORS

RUJUTA A. KATKAR, BDS, MDS, MS
Assistant Professor, Department of Comprehensive Dentistry, University of Texas Health San Antonio, School of Dentistry, San Antonio, Texas, USA

HASSEM GEHA, DDS, MDS
Associate Professor, Division of Oral and Maxillofacial Radiology, Department of Comprehensive Dentistry, University of Texas Health San Antonio, School of Dentistry, San Antonio, Texas, USA

AUTHORS

WISAM AL-RAWI, DDS, MS
Private Practice, Horizon Dental, San Diego, California, USA

BENNETT T. AMAECHI, BDS, MSc, PhD, MFDS RCPS (Glasg), FADI
Professor and Director of Cariology, Department of Comprehensive Dentistry, University of Texas Health San Antonio, School of Dentistry, San Antonio, Texas, USA

CHRISTOS ANGELOPOULOS, DDS, MS
Aristotle University of Thessaloniki, Greece and Columbia University, College of Dental Medicine, Greece

ERIKA BENAVIDES, DDS, PhD
Clinical Associate Professor, Department of Periodontics and Oral Medicine, University of Michigan School of Dentistry, Ann Arbor, Michigan, USA

DOUGLAS K. BENN, DDS, PhD
Professor, Department of Diagnostic Sciences, Creighton University School of Dentistry, Omaha, Nebraska, USA

PATRICK M. COLLETTI, MD
Professor, Department of Radiology, Keck School of Medicine of USC, Los Angeles, California, USA

HUSNIYE DEMIRTURK KOCASARAC, DDS, PhD
Division of Oral and Maxillofacial Radiology, Department of Comprehensive Dentistry, University of Texas Health San Antonio, San Antonio, Texas, USA

DANIEL FRIED, PhD
Professor, Division of Biomaterials and Bioengineering, Department of Preventive and Restorative Dental Sciences, University of California, San Francisco, San Francisco, California, USA

LAURENCE R. GAALAAS, DDS, MS
Clinical Assistant Professor, Oral and Maxillofacial Radiology, Division of Oral Medicine, Diagnosis and Radiology, Department of Diagnostic and Biological Sciences, School of Dentistry, University of Minnesota, Minneapolis, Minnesota, USA

HASSEM GEHA, DDS, MDS
Associate Professor, Division of Oral and Maxillofacial Radiology, Department of Comprehensive Dentistry, University of Texas Health San Antonio, School of Dentistry, San Antonio, Texas, USA

ANITA GOHEL, BDS, PhD
Clinical Professor and Program Director, Oral and Maxillofacial Pathology and Radiology, College of Dentistry, The Ohio State University, Columbus, Ohio, USA

GERALD T. GRANT, DMD, MS, FACP, FAAMP
Professor, Interim Chair, Oral Health and Rehabilitation, University of Louisville School of Dentistry, Louisville, Kentucky, USA

NICOLE HERNANDEZ, DDS, MD
PGY-4, Department of Oral and Maxillofacial Surgery, University of Texas Health San Antonio, Center for Oral Health Care and Research, San Antonio, Texas, USA

AMOL S. KATKAR, MD
Clinical Radiologist, Department of Radiology, Brook Army Medical Center, Fort Sam Houston, Texas, USA

RUJUTA A. KATKAR, BDS, MDS, MS
Assistant Professor, Department of Comprehensive Dentistry, University of Texas Health San Antonio, School of Dentistry, San Antonio, Texas, USA

CARLOS G. LANDAETA-QUINONES, DDS
Faculty, Department of Oral and Maxillofacial Surgery, University of Texas Health San Antonio, Center for Oral Health Care and Research, San Antonio, Texas, USA

ANDRÉ MOL, DDS, MS, PhD
Clinical Associate Professor, Department of Diagnostic Sciences, School of Dentistry, University of North Carolina at Chapel Hill, Chapel Hill, North Carolina, USA

IBRAHIM NASSEH, DDS, DSO
Department of Oral and Maxillofacial Radiology, Lebanese University, School of Dentistry, Beirut, Lebanon

DONALD R. NIXDORF, DDS, MS
Associate Professor, Director, Division of TMD and Orofacial Pain, Department of Diagnostic and Biological Sciences, School of Dentistry, University of Minnesota, Minneapolis, Minnesota, USA

MASAFUMI ODA, DDS, PhD
Research Scholar, Department of Radiology, Boston Medical Center, Boston University School of Medicine, Boston, Massachusetts, USA; Assistant Professor, Division of Oral and Maxillofacial Radiology, Kyushu Dental University, Kitakyushu, Japan

ADEPITAN A. OWOSHO, BChD
Diplomate, American Board of Oral and Maxillofacial Pathology; Fellow, American Academy of Oral Medicine, Edmonds, Washington, USA; Assistant Clinical Professor, Oral and Maxillofacial Pathology and Oral Medicine, College of Dental Medicine, University of New England, Portland, Maine, USA

OSAMU SAKAI, MD, PhD
Chief of Neuroradiology, Professor of Radiology, Departments of Radiology,
Otolaryngology–Head and Neck Surgery and Radiation Oncology, Boston Medical
Center, Boston University School of Medicine, Boston, Massachusetts, USA

SATYASHANKARA ADITYA TADINADA, BDS, MDentSci
Assistant Professor, Oral Health and Diagnostic Sciences, UConn Health, Farmington,
Connecticut, USA

ROBERT M. TAFT, DDS, FACP
Professor, Chairman, Department of Comprehensive Dentistry, University of Texas Health
San Antonio, School of Dentistry, San Antonio, Texas, USA

HEIDI R. WASSEF, MD
Assistant Professor of Clinical Radiology, Department of Radiology, Keck School of
Medicine of USC, PET Center, Los Angeles, California, USA

DOUGLAS C. YOON, DDS
President/Chief Technology Officer, Research and Development, XDR Radiology,
Los Angeles, California, USA

NAJY K. ZARROUG, DDS, MD
PGY-6, Department of Oral and Maxillofacial Surgery, University of Texas Health
San Antonio, Center for Oral Health Care and Research, San Antonio, Texas, USA

Contents

temporomandibular joint surgery, facial trauma, maxillomandibular reconstruction, implantology, and restorative dentistry. This article describes the indications of CAS in dentistry and CMF; reviews the process, benefits, and shortcomings; and discusses the future of CAS.

Rujuta A. Katkar, Satyashankara Aditya Tadinada, Bennett T. Amaechi, and Daniel Fried

Optical coherence tomography (OCT) is a noninvasive diagnostic technique providing cross-sectional images of biologic structures based on the differences in tissue optical properties. OCT has been widely used in numerous clinical applications and is becoming popular as a promising technology in dentistry. Today, dental hard (tooth) and soft (hard palate mucosa and gingiva mucosa) tissues are visualized with OCT. With new developments in technology, the applications of OCT are being investigated in various fields in dentistry, such as detection of microleakage around restoration and tooth cracks/fractures, examination of periodontal tissues/pockets, early detection of oral cancerous tissues, and in endodontics for location of pulp canal.

Bennett T. Amaechi, Adepitan A. Owosho, and Daniel Fried

This article describes the current applications of various technologies based on either autofluorescence or near-infrared light illumination, tailored to aid practitioners in detecting and quantitatively monitoring oral diseases, such as dental caries and oral cancer, at the earliest stage of their formation or in the conservative surgical excision of necrotic bones in diseases such as chronic osteomyelitis, osteoradionecrosis, and medication-related osteonecrosis of the jaw. The data discussed are primarily based on published scientific studies and reviews from case reports, clinical trials, and in vitro and in vivo studies. References have been traced manually, by MEDLINE, or through manufacturer's websites.

Anita Gohel, Masafumi Oda, Amol S. Katkar, and Osamu Sakai

Multidetector row computed tomography (MDCT) offers superior soft tissue characterization and is useful for the diagnosis of odontogenic and nonodontogenic cysts and tumors; fibroosseous lesions; inflammatory, malignant, and metastatic lesions; developmental abnormalities; and maxillofacial trauma. The rapid advances in MDCT technology, including perfusion CT, dual-energy CT, and texture analysis, will be an integrated anatomic and functional high-resolution scan, which will help in the diagnosis of maxillofacial lesions and overall patient care.

Husniye Demirturk Kocasarac, Hassem Geha, Laurence R. Gaalaas, and Donald R. Nixdorf

Imaging of hard and soft tissue of the oral cavity is important for dentistry. However, medical computed tomography, cone beam computed tomography (CBCT), or MRI do not enable soft and hard tissue imaging simultaneously. Some MRI sequences were shown to provide fast soft and hard tissue imaging of hydrogen, which increased the interest in dental MRI. Recently, MRI allowed direct visualization of cancellous bone, intraoral mucosa, and dental pulp despite that cortical bone and dental roots are indirectly visualized. MRI seems to be adequate for many indications that CBCT is currently used for: implant treatment and inflammatory diseases of the tooth.

Ultrasonography (US) is a noninvasive, nonionizing, inexpensive, and painless imaging tool proven to be a valuable diagnostic tool in soft tissue assessment that also shows promise for hard tissue evaluation in dentistry. US has been investigated for its capability to identify carious lesions, tooth fractures or cracks, periodontal bony defects, maxillofacial fractures, and more. It has been used as a diagnostic aid in temporomandibular disorders, in implant dentistry, and to measure muscle and soft tissue thickness. Unfortunately, the use of US in dentistry is still in its infancy; however, relevant research is promising.

Nuclear medicine studies evaluate physiology on a molecular level, providing earlier detection of lesions before morphologic change is evident. ^{99m}Tc-MDP and ^{18}F-fluoride bone scans detect osteomyelitis earlier than radiography and computed tomography (CT); aid in the diagnosis of temporomandibular joint disorder; and evaluate the activity of condylar hyperplasia, extent of Paget disease, and viability of bone grafts. ^{18}F-FDG PET/CT distinguish between soft tissue and bone infections and diagnose osteomyelitis complicated by fracture or surgery. FDG PET is more accurate than CT alone and has a major role in staging, restaging, and assessing response to therapy for head and neck malignancies and in detecting sequelae of therapy.

Preface

Emerging Imaging Technologies in Dentomaxillofacial Radiology

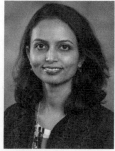

Rujuta A. Kalkar, BDS, MDS, MS   Hassem Geha, DDS, MDS
Editors

Keeping up with emerging technologies is vital for the survival and growth of any profession. Technology is ever advancing in today's world, and if you don't keep up with it, you run a risk of falling behind and even becoming irrelevant. As with every other profession, dentistry has embraced the latest technological advances in all of its specialties. With better understanding and integration of physics and computer science, imaging in the dentomaxillofacial region is not limited to the use of radiographs anymore. Fluorescence, thermal imaging, and near-infrared imaging are being explored for caries detection. MRI, ultrasound, and optical coherence tomography have been around for a while, but recent research shows promise for their use in dentistry. Advanced digital technology has facilitated the integration of computed tomography scan data in techniques such as 3D printing and computer-assisted navigational surgery.

The purpose of this publication is to update dental professionals, especially oral and maxillofacial radiologists, on the emerging imaging technologies, which they are already using or potentially going to encounter in the near future. The emphasis of the articles is on the latest developments in various imaging techniques in the dentomaxillofacial region.

The articles are outlined and arranged from the most to the least commonly used technologies in dentistry, such that every article sets the stage for the following one and the end result would be comprehensible to the reader. The opening article is on digital radiographic image processing and analysis that spans from the basics of image capture to examples of some of the most advanced digital technologies currently available, including artificial intelligence. The authors have described the principles underlying the imaging technologies to provide a better understanding of their strengths and

Dent Clin N Am 62 (2018) xi–xii
https://doi.org/10.1016/j.cden.2018.04.001
0011-8532/18/© 2018 Published by Elsevier Inc.

limitations. It is followed by articles on cone beam computed tomography and 3D printing. Other articles discuss the process, benefits, and shortcomings of computer-assisted (navigational) surgery. Two articles follow, one on optical coherence tomography and the other on fluorescence and near-infrared imaging, which appear promising in the field of caries detection. Technologies that are more frequently used in the medical field than in the dental field are covered in the final part of the current issue, discussing updates in multidetector computed tomography, MRI, ultrasonography, and nuclear medicine.

We are grateful to all the renowned authors who were instrumental in creating this issue of *Dental Clinics of North America*. We hope that their work will stimulate interest in the readers and will inspire further research in the field of the dentomaxillofacial region.

Rujuta A. Katkar, BDS, MDS, MS
Department of Comprehensive Dentistry
University of Texas Health San Antonio
School of Dentistry
7703 Floyd Curl Drive
San Antonio, TX 78229, USA

Hassem Geha, DDS, MDS
Department of Comprehensive Dentistry
University of Texas Health San Antonio
School of Dentistry
7703 Floyd Curl Drive
San Antonio, TX 78229, USA

E-mail addresses:
katkarR@uthscsa.edu (R.A. Katkar)
geha@uthscsa.edu (H. Geha)

Digital Radiographic Image Processing and Analysis

Douglas C. Yoon, DDS[a],*, André Mol, DDS, MS, PhD[b], Douglas K. Benn, DDS, PhD[c], Erika Benavides, DDS, PhD[d]

KEYWORDS

- Image processing • Digital imaging • Image analysis • Tomosynthesis
- Artificial intelligence • Conebeam • Image processing artifacts • Image recognition

KEY POINTS

- Image processing, although useful in accentuating diagnostic features, has the potential to mimic or hide clinical pathosis. The clinician should always refer to the original image to confirm diagnosis.
- Reconstruction adds valuable information by combining multiple views.
- Artificial intelligence programs perform complex tasks normally associated with human brains. Dental examples could be the identification and reporting of image artifacts that could produce false disease changes. Seeing is controlled hallucination.
- Advanced imaging and image processing is not always precise and may introduce artifacts, always requiring the use of clinical judgment.

INTRODUCTION

Twenty years ago an article on this subject would not be found in a clinical dentistry textbook but today it would be remiss to not include such an article. The reason for this change is the almost complete transition from film-based imaging to digital-based image capture and display. In fact, it is quite possible that some of the younger generation of dental clinicians today may never have taken a film-based radiograph.

Disclosure Statement: Dr D.C. Yoon is CTO and founder of XDR Radiology. Dr A. Mol is a coinventor of intraoral tomosynthesis using a carbon nanotube–based field emission X-ray source and is on the Board of Advisors of XinVivo, Inc.

[a] Research and Development, XDR Radiology, 11300 West Olympic Boulevard, Suite 710, Los Angeles, CA 90064, USA; [b] Department of Diagnostic Sciences, School of Dentistry, University of North Carolina at Chapel Hill, 385 South Columbia Street, Chapel Hill, NC 27599, USA; [c] Department of Diagnostic Sciences, Creighton University School of Dentistry, 2802 Webster Street, Omaha, NE 68178, USA; [d] Department of Periodontics and Oral Medicine, University of Michigan School of Dentistry, 2029F, 1011 North University Avenue, Ann Arbor, MI 49109-1078, USA
* Corresponding author.
E-mail address: dyoon@XDRemail.com

Although the imagery generated by the two modalities may look the same, the technical aspects could not be more different and these differences have significant clinical consequences. The purpose of this article is to give the reader a basic understanding of digital imaging, in both its power and limitations, and discuss recent advances in this technology.

It is useful to start with a brief discussion of film-based radiography, which is still a powerful imaging modality and considered by some the standard by which the newer technologies are compared. Unlike digital imaging, film-based radiography is a physically intuitive and understandable technology that allows the clinician to monitor and control almost every step of the process. In addition, once a radiograph is produced, it remains as a physical object that for all practical purposes is unalterable. Changing the ambient room lighting or the strength of the backlighting are the only means to compensate for underexposure or overexposure. Also, film is a negative image; that is, a high level of radiant energy makes the film image dark, whereas the raw digital image is light when it absorbs a high level of radiant energy. The image intensity is inverted in digital imagery only to make the image look like film; such is the strong heritage of film.

By comparison, digital radiography is not physically intuitive or easily monitored at every step of the process because most of the processing is hidden in algorithms implemented in electronics. Also, the radiograph is not a fixed physical object. Rather, the radiograph is only seen as a temporary display on a computer screen and produced from invisible digital data originally captured by solid-state electronic sensors or phosphor plate scanners. The appearance of this display can be easily modified by the software algorithms presenting the radiograph, making it difficult for the clinician to trace the pedigree of a digital radiograph. Even more important, some of these algorithms may produce artifacts that affect diagnosis. This last fact may present serious clinical and legal challenges.

The following sections describe step by step the image capture and display process, including the capabilities and potential hazards. The capabilities derive from the power of modern high-speed computers to quickly manipulate large quantities of data and the potential hazards come from the ability to easily perform inappropriate processing and analysis.

Composition of an Image

The most basic definition of an image, for purposes of this discussion, is a spatial array of different brightness levels at each location in the array. For a film image, the brightness or density at any location in the image are determined by the density of silver crystals at that location. The distribution of these crystals is random and disorganized (**Fig. 1**A). By comparison, digital image brightness values are defined at specific locations on a highly organized rectangular grid in units called pixels (picture elements). The position of each pixel is uniquely specified by its horizontal and vertical location within the grid (**Fig. 1**B). The more pixels an image contains, the more image data can be shown. Also, the smaller the size of a pixel, the smaller the details the image can display. Note that for 3-dimensional (3D) imagery, the equivalent of a pixel is called a voxel (volume element). The number of pixels and the size of each pixel are determined by the structure of the sensor that captured the image.

Image Capture

Most digital radiographic intraoral and extraoral imagery are captured by solid-state devices, similar to the charge-coupled device (CCD) and complementary metal-oxide semiconductor (CMOS) or thin-film transistor (TFT) devices one might find in

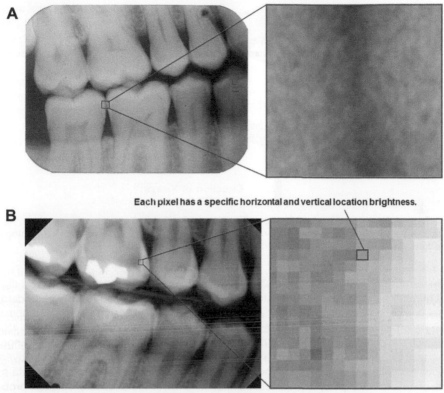

Fig. 1. (*A*) A film image consists of many randomly placed and irregularly shaped silver crystals. The image density is proportional to the crystal size and crystal density. (*B*) A digital image consists of a uniform array of pixels. A pixel is specified by its horizontal and vertical location and a brightness value.

cell phones, cameras, and displays; the exception is photostimulable phosphor (PSP) plate systems. For radiography, these CCD and CMOS or TFT devices are modified to capture X-ray photons instead of visible light photons. **Fig. 2** shows an expanded view of a typical CMOS intraoral imaging sensor. Note that the addition of a scintillator layer allows such devices to form visible light images from X-ray energy.

Solid-state imaging devices consist of rectangular arrays of many individual detectors, in which each detector corresponds to a pixel in the image and the size of the detector is essentially the physical size of the pixel. Pixels are usually square and typical dimensions are 15 to 40 microns squared. During operation, when X-ray photons are absorbed in the scintillator layer, visible light photons are produced and transmitted to the CMOS visible light imager. Within the CMOS imager, the visible light photons produce an electric charge within each pixel, which is then amplified and converted to an equivalent voltage that is proportional to the number of photons intercepted by the pixel. Hence, pixels with higher voltage represent regions of the image with greater radiographic density, similar to film. The voltage level from each pixel is converted to a digitized value that is uploaded to the host computer. The host computer receives these numbers in an organized digital stream that is ready for further processing and display. **Fig. 3** is a generic illustration of the multistep image capture process and how, at each step, the information is slightly degraded.

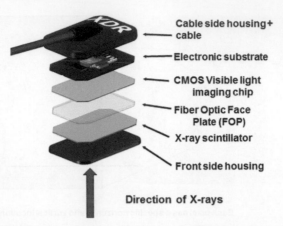

Cable side housing +
cable

Electronic substrate

CMOS Visible light
imaging chip

Fiber Optic Face
Plate (FOP)

X-ray scintillator

Front side housing

Direction of X-rays

Fig. 2. A typical digital intraoral sensor. The X-ray scintillator creates a visible light image that can be captured by a conventional CMOS imaging chip. (*Courtesy of* XDR Radiology, Los Angeles, CA.)

In the context of this article, it is useful to view the conversion from voltages to a digital number as the first and most fundamental processing applied to the image data. This is also called analog-to-digital conversion (ADC). Problems with this process can have serious clinical consequences. The most serious is data clipping (**Fig. 4**B), in which the pixel output voltage is higher than the upper limit of the digitization range. This might happen when the X-ray exposure is too high. All density information in overexposed regions would be lost. The engineering solution is to allocate more data or bits of data to each pixel. The clinical solution is to lower the exposure. Another problem is insufficient resolution of digitization. In this case, too few digits of precision are allocated to encode the output pixel voltage levels, resulting in abrupt changes in brightness along what should be smooth density gradients. This effect is called posterization. This effect could cause one to miss subtle lesions. Again, the engineering solution is to allocate more data or bits per pixel. The clinical solution is to extend the pixel output voltage range by increasing the exposure (however, care should be taken not to go beyond the recommended exposure guidelines or to cause data clipping). Problems with ADC can be subtle and different from film but important for the clinician to recognize. Fortunately, problems with ADC are rare because the sensor

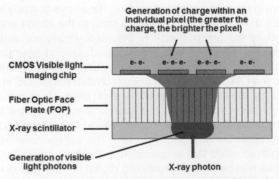

Generation of charge within an
individual pixel (the greater the
charge, the brighter the pixel)

CMOS Visible light
imaging chip

Fiber Optic Face
Plate (FOP)

X-ray scintillator

Generation of visible
light photons

X-ray photon

Fig. 3. Conceptual diagram showing the image capture process (not drawn to scale). Each stage induces additional beam spread (*red*), which causes blurring.

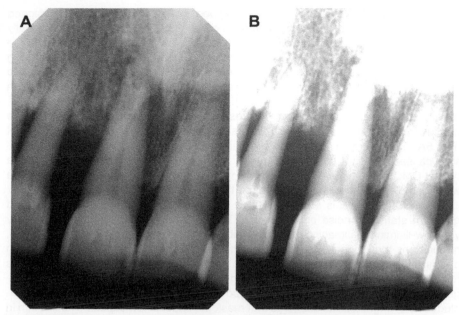

Fig. 4. (A) Original image with no selective contrast treatment. (B) Same image with selective accentuation of the darker portions of the image. Note the greater visualization of the crestal bone and gingiva but the loss of detail in the brighter regions of the image (an example of data clipping).

engineers carefully consider these factors when designing the hardware and control software.

Over the last several years, advancements in sensor technology have been evolutionary rather than revolutionary, which is characteristic for the semiconductor industry as a whole. Some of the advancements include a transition from CCD to CMOS architecture and more efficient scintillators, as well as improved ergonomics. The newer generation sensors exhibit greater sensitivity and resolution, lower noise and power consumption, have simpler computer interfaces, and are more comfortable for the patient. The authors know no reason for these trends not to continue in the future.

Image Processing

Because of the ADC process, the image data are readily available and specified on a rectangular grid. All the image processing applications are readily available to the clinician using image viewing software. Today's computers can perform billions of operations per second, allowing for the implementation of sophisticated processing and display algorithms unheard of just a few years ago. The computer and imaging software render the data in a form that is recognizable as a radiograph on a computer display. This following section gives a brief overview of the types of computer-based image processing currently available. It proceeds from the most basic, low-level data processing to the most advanced. This technology continues to advance at a rapid rate.

Data calibration

Data calibration is the lowest level processing applied to the raw image data as it comes off the ADC from the acquisition device (eg, CCD, CMOS, TFT, PSP). Most users are not aware of this level of processing because these algorithms are designed to compensate for the engineering limitations of the capture hardware and are usually automatically applied at the time of image capture. These include algorithms to reduce electronic noise. Because this type of noise tends to form consistent patterns among the pixels, it is often termed patterned noise. As such, these effects are often easy to correct for, using what is often called calibration data (or file). Each sensor has its own characteristic fixed noise pattern, so calibration data files are not interchangeable. Also, it is important to recognize the presence of excessive fixed patterned noise because it can also indicate electronic failure or an extremely low exposure level (**Fig. 5**A). This example shows patterned electronic noise associated with low exposure caused by slight differences in gain between different column amplifiers in a typical CMOS image resulting in streaks in the image. **Fig. 5**B shows the same data with a simple algorithm applied to reduce this effect.

Unfortunately, there is a form of noise that is difficult to compensate for called quantum statistical noise or shot noise. This is because radiography is basically very low-illumination imaging. Like low visible light images (eg, night-vision imaging), radiographs tend to look speckled or grainy (see **Fig. 5**A). This effect has no pattern and is difficult to compensate for without reducing image sharpness. The authors mention this type of noise because among the most common causes of poor radiographic quality for digital is insufficient exposure. Digital image processing usually includes auto-brightness adjustments that mask the effect of low exposure (unlike film in which an underexposed image would look too light and washed out). An increased grainy pattern may be the only indication of low exposure.

Brightness and contrast adjustments

Beyond calibration, there are processing algorithms to change the overall brightness and contrast of the image. These types of processes give the user control over the radiographic appearance not possible for film radiography. They involve a simple reassignment of the pixel brightness in the digitized data from the original image. This is accomplished by algorithms to assign new brightness values to each pixel with a

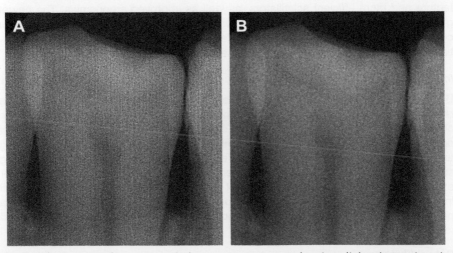

Fig. 5. (A) Close-up of an extremely low exposure image showing slight electronic noise (vertical stripes). (B) Same image with electronic noise-reduction treatment. Both images show graininess due to shot noise.

simple treatment of the data. This treatment is controlled by the user with the imaging software and determines the final appearance of the radiograph. The same treatment is applied to all pixels independently, hence, if the exact nature of the treatment is known, then the alteration may be reversed, if the change is not so extreme as to cause posterization (see previous discussion) when reversed. Because these treatments alter the distribution of pixel intensities, these are also called histogram manipulations (**Fig. 6**A).

The simplest example of these histogram manipulations is the histogram stretch. The purpose of this procedure is to increase the dynamic range of the image to cover the full brightness range of the display on the monitor (usually 0–255). To provide sufficient exposure latitude, the dynamic range of the raw data is almost always significantly less than the maximum possible. Thus, some kind of stretch of the output is needed to present a clinically diagnostic image. **Fig. 6**B and C show an example of this type of data treatment. Note the low overall contrast of the raw data. This is characteristic of all solid-state image capture devices. However, clinically, this can make the perception of subtle radiolucencies or subtle soft tissue structures difficult.

This illustrates an advantage of digital radiography over film. One can dynamically apply different brightness assignment treatments, allowing the user to selectively stretch the brightness range of only a portion of the entire density range of a radiograph. For example, when looking for details in soft tissue structures, the clinician can stretch the brightness range of the image only in the dark portions of the image where one would expect to see soft tissue structures (**Fig. 4**). However, as this example illustrates, if one portion of the brightness range is stretched, detail is lost at other brightness levels (in this example, the lighter portions of the image). Thus, to preserve the original image data, it is important to always store the raw data from the sensors. Brightness or contrast adjustments always destroy or degrade data, therefore such adjustments should always be done for display purposes only and

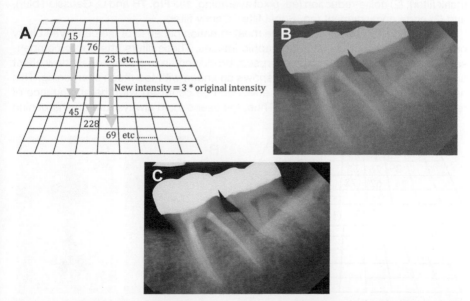

New intensity = 3 * original intensity

Fig. 6. (*A*) A simple histogram manipulation. The original brightness of each pixel is multiplied by 3. (*B*) Original untreated image. (*C*) Treated image. This expands the dynamic range of the image, improving overall contrast.

the image processing and analysis software should always go back to the original raw data. Also, the user should learn to recognize when such adjustments have been applied. Terms such as gamma, sigmoid, exponential, and logarithmic treatments are just examples of the different types of brightness assignment treatments that vendors use in their imaging software. The user should try all the different treatments to learn their effects on clinical images.

Before concluding this section, it should be mentioned that it is possible to convert brightness values to different colors. This is often referred to as colorization and it produces esthetically interesting images but it has little clinical value and is not discussed further.[1]

Image filters

The term image filter loosely applies to a class of image processing that involves the use of more sophisticated algorithms than simple histogram manipulations. Whereas the latter acts independently on each pixel, filters often involve complex interactions between pixels, usually groups of neighboring pixels (**Fig. 7**A). This mathematical interaction creates a complexity that often makes the resulting images quite different from the original, sensitive to image noise, prone to artifact production, and irreversible in operation. However, this complexity, if properly and carefully applied, has the potential to elucidate subtle features in the image far beyond simple histogram manipulations. Most of the filters in this category are designed to either affect spatial resolution, which is defined as the ability to distinguish closely spaced objects in an image, or to affect contrast perceptibility, which is the ability to distinguish subtle changes in intensity or radiographic density.

By far, the most common types of mathematical operations in this class are image convolutions (and deconvolutions) in which the image is mathematically convolved with a filter (or kernel); hence the name image filter. There are many types of filters designed to perform a variety of functions. These include (1) sharpening (eg, unsharp mask filter), (2) noise-reduction (eg, pixel averaging; see **Fig. 7**B and C, Gaussian blur), and (3) edge enhancement (eg, Sobel filter, Canny filter).

Sharpening filters have received the most attention because of the perceived blurry or soft appearance of digital radiographic images. These filters attempt to compensate for this effect but tend to be overused, producing an overshoot or shadow effect around bright restorations.[2-4] **Fig. 8** shows an image with too much sharpening. This has clinical significance because its effect can be confused with the appearance of recurrent decay under restorations. Thus, the user should always turn off sharpening

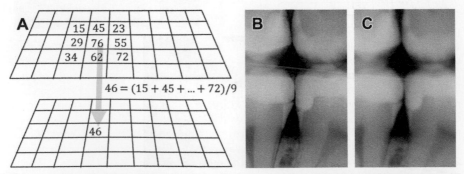

Fig. 7. (A) Advanced image filter. Each pixel is assigned the average of itself and its 8 neighbors. (B) Original unfiltered image. (C) Averaging filtered image. Note reduction in noise but loss of detail.

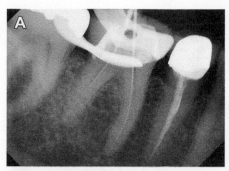 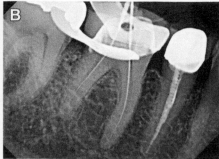

Fig. 8. (*A*) Original untreated image, (*B*) Oversharpened image. Note dark halo around the rubber dam clamp and restorations. Such an effect around restorations may be confused with recurrent decay.

filters when attempting to confirm the presence of any pathosis. In addition, sharpening filters are highly sensitive to the presence of image noise; that is, they can accentuate the random variations in image intensity.

Noise-reduction filters, such as averaging filters (see **Fig. 7**) and Gaussian blur, accomplish the opposite of sharpening filters; that is, image detail is reduced while reducing noise. This is accomplished by spreading out the intensity of a pixel to its surrounding neighbors. These filters are often applied for aesthetic reasons and there is no clinical evidence that these filters enhance diagnosis.[5] Whenever the clinician sees excessively smooth images, they should suspect excessive blurring and loss of potentially diagnostic spatial details.

Geometric correction

To a limited extent, actual correction for geometry and not just length scaling (see later discussion) can be applied to 2-dimensional (2D) intraoral imagery if some type of X-ray beam orientation reference is in the image that indicates the direction of the X-ray beam relative to the sensor. **Fig. 9** shows an example of the type of digital correction that can be applied to an image. Note the elongation of the spherical reference object. The image has been corrected to represent the image that would be produced if perfect paralleling technique were applied at image capture. Such algorithms cannot correct for foreshortening of the subject, which are considered irreversible.[6]

Image reconstruction

The integration of imaging and computer technology has enabled the development of new imaging modalities based on image reconstruction. Image reconstruction, sometimes referred to as image synthesis, creates an image not through direct acquisition but rather through computational methods that reconstruct or synthesize other projection images or nonimage data. Generally, the main purpose is to provide 3D information about the patient. When projection images (**Fig. 10**A) are used as the basis for reconstructing new images, the level of 3D information is determined by the angular disparity between the different projections (ie, basis projections). The quality of the reconstructed image is, in part, determined by the number of basis projections.

In its most elementary form, image reconstruction can be performed with only 2 basis images. Digital subtraction radiography is based on the registration of 2 basis projections with identical projection geometry; that is, with zero degrees of angular disparity (**Fig. 10**B). Therefore, there is no true 3D information in subtraction images. When 2 basis projections are acquired with a small angular disparity, a stereoscopic

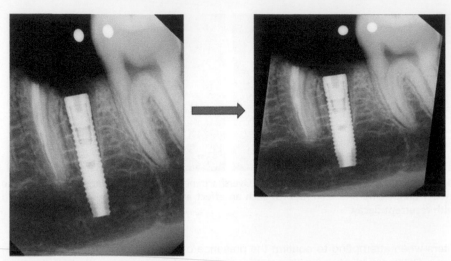

Fig. 9. Example of correction for image distortion due to tilting of the sensor relative to the X-ray beam. (*Right*) The original radiograph, showing extreme elongation of all objects in radiograph, including a spherical reference. (*Left*) Geometrically corrected image. Note the change in length and the restored shape of the spherical reference. (*Courtesy of* XDR Radiology, Los Angeles, CA.)

view can be generated (**Fig. 10**C). The 2 projections are not actually used to reconstruct a new image. Instead they are viewed side-by side, either with the aid of a stereoscope or with trained eyes, allowing a limited amount of depth perception by the viewer. When more than 2 basis projections are generated with increasing but still limited angular disparity, tomosynthetic images can be reconstructed (**Fig. 10**D). In tomosynthesis, thin image slices are reconstructed in a plane parallel to the detector, which allows visualization of structures in a single plane without superimposition of structures in another plane. This imaging technique is not new and dental applications were developed 2 decades ago. The clinical implementation of tomosynthesis stalled at that time because of the cumbersome acquisition protocols, time-consuming reconstruction techniques, and the introduction of dental conebeam computed tomography (CBCT). A resurgent interest in tomosynthesis has been seen in recent years with the development of tomosynthesis-based panoramic radiography and the development of carbon nanotube (CNT)-based field emission X-ray sources for intraoral tomosynthesis (see later discussion).

The acquisition of a large number of basis projections with an angular disparity of at least 180° is able to resolve complete 3D information through the reconstruction of an image volume (**Fig. 10**E). Traditionally, multidetector computed tomography (MDCT) scanners use multiple 360-degree rotations of a fan-beam X-ray source and a narrow detector. (See Anita Gohel and colleagues' article, "MDCT in Maxillofacial Imaging," in this issue.) CBCT scanners use a single rotation between 180° and 360° of a conventional X-ray source and an area detector. The word conebeam is a misnomer now because the beam is collimated to a rectangular pyramidal shape to match the dimensions of the rectangular flat panel detector (see later discussion). (See Ibrahim Nasseh and Wisam Al-Rawi's article, "Cone Beam Computed Tomography," in this issue.) An example of a 3D image reconstruction technology that is based on nonimage data is MRI. This modality relies on the detection of resonant radiofrequency signals from the patient in the presence of a strong magnetic field. (See Husniye Demirturk Kocasarac

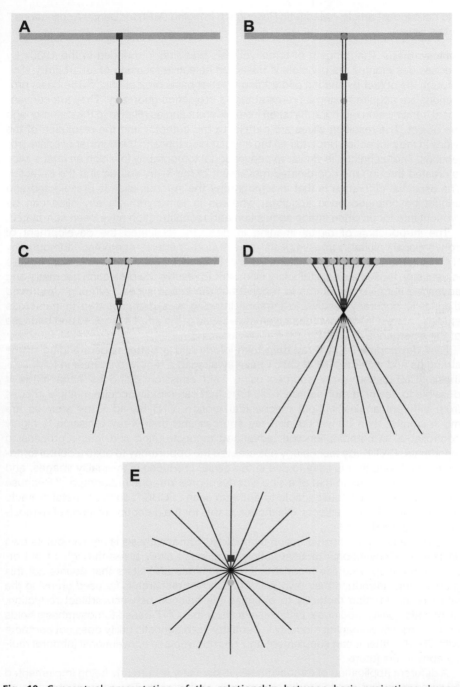

Fig. 10. Conceptual presentation of the relationship between basis projections, image reconstruction, and the ability to resolve 3D information. (*A*) Transmission radiography. (*B*) Digital subtraction radiography. (*C*) Stereoscopic radiography. (*D*) Tomosynthesis. (*E*) Computed tomography (multidetector computed tomography and conebeam computed tomography).

and colleagues' article, "Magnetic Resonance Imaging (MRI) for Dental Applications," in this issue.)

Tomosynthesis The concept of tomosynthesis was first introduced in the 1930s by Ziedses des Plantes. Its principle is based on selective focusing of an arbitrary slice through the object by shifting and adding a set of basis projections.[7,8] The basis projections are acquired using a pre-established projection geometry. They are conventional transmission radiographs taken from different angles relative to the detector and the object. The resulting slices are parallel to the detector and the resolution of the slices in the z-direction depends on the angular disparity and the number of basis projections. The technique is similar to conventional tomography in which an image slice is created through the coordinated movement of the X-ray source and the detector. The essential difference is that in tomography the in-focus slice is preselected and cannot be changed once acquired, whereas in tomosynthesis any slice can be brought into focus when image acquisition and reconstruction have been completed.

The introduction of digital imaging in dentistry facilitated the development of conventional digital tomosynthesis and tuned-aperture computed tomography (TACT). In the 1990s, TACT became the most advanced application of tomosynthesis in dentistry. It used a single fiduciary landmark to resolve the projection geometry and advanced iterative algorithms to reconstruct the image slices.[9] Although improved diagnostic accuracy relative to intraoral imaging was demonstrated in numerous studies, interest in tomosynthesis waned because of the effort it required and because of the emergence of CBCT.

New developments in X-ray tube technology and a better understanding of the strengths and weaknesses of CBCT have awakened a renewed interest in tomosynthesis. CNT-based X-ray sources using field emission cathodes have made it possible to design a multisource X-ray tube that can rapidly acquire multiple images from different angles without mechanical motion. CNT-based X-ray sources are much smaller than conventional X-ray sources and their X-ray emission is highly controllable. In combination with advanced reconstruction and image processing algorithms, CNT X-ray technology has created the opportunity to build a dental tomosynthetic device that is easy to use in the clinic, produces high-quality images, and limits the dose close to that of a single conventional intraoral radiograph.[10] Because tomosynthesis is less susceptible to artifacts seen in CBCT, such as metal artifacts and beam-hardening artifacts, it is more suitable for the detection of signs of dentoalveolar disease (**Fig. 11**).

As with any image reconstruction technology, tomosynthesis is not without its own limitations. Conventional reconstruction techniques allow bleed-through of out-of-focus structures, whereas reconstruction algorithms and filters that counteract this problem may introduce their own artifacts. Current research is focused on using the latest reconstruction methods to optimize the balance between artifact reduction, diagnostic quality, and dose. Initial results show that CNT-based tomosynthesis holds promise as a new imaging modality in dentistry. Its diagnostic utility does not compete with CBCT, rather it can supplement and possibly replace conventional intraoral radiography in the future.

A different application of tomosynthesis in dentistry is currently being implemented by some manufactures to produce panoramic radiographs. The concept of tomosynthetic panoramic radiography is not new.[11] Similar to intraoral tomosynthesis, a panoramic unit can acquire multiple nontomographic images during 1 rotation instead of 1 single tomographic image. The advantage of the tomosynthetic approach is the ability to focus and refocus the image layer after acquisition.

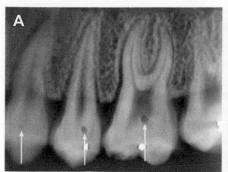 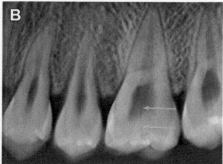

Fig. 11. Two tomosynthetic slices of the same object. (A) The buccal roots of the first molar and simulated caries lesions (*yellow arrows*). (B) The palatal root of the first molar and a fracture line (*green arrows*).

Conebeam computed tomography Computed tomography is a classic example of a reconstruction imaging modality. Both MDCT and CBCT rely on the reconstruction of volume data based on the acquisition of 2D X-ray projections. In CBCT, those projections consist of a series of basis projections, some of which are very similar to traditional lateral and posteroanterior cephalometric radiographs. With the addition of a large number of projections between those orthogonal views, algorithms are used to compute the attenuation characteristics of small areas within the patient and reconstruct the patient's anatomy in 3D. Reconstruction algorithms that are commonly used are either based on analytical methods, such as filtered back-projection, or on iterative methods, such as the algebraic reconstruction technique. The former is efficient but prone to produce artifacts in the presence of complicating factors such as metal. The latter is computationally more demanding (ie, less efficient) but is more versatile and generally produces images with fewer artifacts. Regardless of the algorithm, CBCT volume reconstruction remains an exercise of estimation and can contain artifacts that have no analog in traditional projection radiography.[12,13] It is imperative for the clinician to be aware of some of those artifacts because they may interfere with disease detection or may induce signals that mimic disease. Artifacts can be categorized as physics-based, patient-based, or scanner-based. Examples of physics-based artifacts include beam hardening, partial volume, and aliasing artifacts. Beam hardening artifacts are inherent in all forms of computed tomography and are the result of classic X-ray attenuation physics. These artifacts are particularly troublesome in dentistry because high-density structures, such as enamel and dental materials, can cause profound beam hardening. As a result, adjacent dentin may show a localized area of low density mimicking caries and an endodontically treated root may show multiple low-density lines mimicking root fractures. Examples of patient-based artifacts include metal and motion artifacts. Whereas fixed metal restorations cannot be removed, motion artifacts can be prevented or minimized by using head restraints, having the patient sit instead of stand, and by using adequate patient instruction. Ring artifacts and conebeam effect artifacts are examples of scanner-based artifacts, among others. Although an in-depth discussion of CBCT artifacts is beyond the scope of this article, minimization of artifacts during image acquisition and recognition of artifacts during interpretation is critical. One of the strengths of CBCT is that, through image reconstruction, the image volume represents the patient's anatomy in a spatially intuitive format. As such, it can deceive the viewer in thinking that the perceived image density values are valid, accurate, and precise, which the reconstruction process cannot guarantee. This underscores the need for adequate training in the use of reconstruction-based imaging and in the interpretation of reconstructed images.

Image Analysis

In addition to image processing that alters the appearance of a radiograph, computer programs can also extract information from images that may aid the clinician in diagnosis and treatment planning. This may range from obtaining simple measurements to advanced interpretive operations. Two examples are given in the following sections.

Measurements: length, density, angle, and so forth

One of the advantages of digital imagery is the ease with which length, relative position, angles, and even the density of objects can be measured in the radiograph. The key to accuracy for all these types of measurements is the presence in the radiograph of a standard reference for the quantity being measured. For example, length measurements require the inclusion of a reference object of known length with a buccal-lingual tilt similar to the object being measured. This allows for correction of geometric distortion, such as magnification, foreshortening, and elongation. The physical size of the sensor and pixels is very stable, so no pixel size calibration is needed. Most so-called calibration is really relating pixel size to the physical size of an object in the radiograph, or length scaling. Measurements made without length references, using only physical pixel size, are equivalent to measuring only the radiographic length and should be used with caution. Using a reference object that is embedded in the detector similarly provides a measure of radiographic size and not actual size.

When dealing with more than one object in the radiograph, the situation becomes even more complex. Although one can try to radiographically measure the relative positions and angles of objects in an intraoral radiograph, the limitations of 2D imaging are severe and the gold standard is 3D volumetric imaging for precise geometric measurements.

For density, again, one needs fiduciaries to obtain absolute rather than relative density measurements. Accurate density measurements are extremely difficult and used primarily in research settings.[14] Simple tools that provide relative density profiles, although interesting, have limited clinical value[15] other than as patient education aids.

Artificial intelligence applications applied to radiography

Seeing is taken for granted. One looks and one sees something. However, seeing is a very complex phenomenon that involves focusing a scene on the retina followed by tremendous computation in the brain where elements of the picture are processed to produce image features such as edges, outlines, and regions. These raw features are then matched against models in the brain. When a pattern of features matches a model of a "thing," we see the "thing." Seeing is in fact a form of controlled hallucination[16] in which one only recognizes what one knows. Hence the need for being taught what radiographic features constitute a "caries tooth thing" and "periodontal bone destruction thing."

Digital image processing changes images so that a human observer can find features easier. However, the recognition or seeing is still performed by the brain. Artificial intelligence (AI) programs are different than image processing because they replace the brain to do the recognition or seeing.

AI can be defined as computer programs that perform complex tasks normally associated with human brain activity, such as interactive speech conversations, recognition of objects in images, disease diagnosis, and planning of treatment. Here, only applications related to images and some possible clinical tasks are discussed. In general, AI programs should try to perform tasks that are too complicated and/or time-consuming for clinicians to routinely perform. In caries management this could be monitoring of posterior interproximal lucency depth and depth change over time because this information is used in conjunction with caries risk assessment to decide when to restore teeth. Ideally, all interproximal lesions should be classified into 5 grades of radiographic depth: outer and inner halves of enamel, or inner-middle-inner thirds of dentin; cavitation state (noncavitated or cavitated); and activity (static or progressing).[17] Evidence-based caries management advises not to restore interproximal enamel lucencies but only cavitated dentin lucencies.[18] A patient with low risk for caries with an outer one-third dentin radiolucency is unlikely to be cavitated and does not need a restoration. A patient with high risk for caries with the same depth radiolucency is likely to be cavitated and needs a restoration.[18] Unfortunately the depth of a radiolucency that appears to be just into dentin with no radiographic overlapping contact surfaces can be projected deeper into outer or middle third dentin with a more oblique X-ray beam direction that causes contact point overlap (**Fig. 12**).[19] This means that variations in X-ray beam direction between different examinations can produce false changes in the apparent depth of a radiolucency. Not only can lesions appear to be deeper but also misinterpreted as progressing with increased caries risk status. For a clinician to decide if a change in depth between examinations is valid or artifactual, the degree of contact point overlap should be compared to see if it has changed. Radiolucency depth changes with constant contact overlap are valid but if the overlap has changed then any radiolucency change should be treated with suspicion.

Evidence-based caries management now requires lesion depth, cavitation state, activity, and risk status to be assessed for every lesion. In addition, the validity of

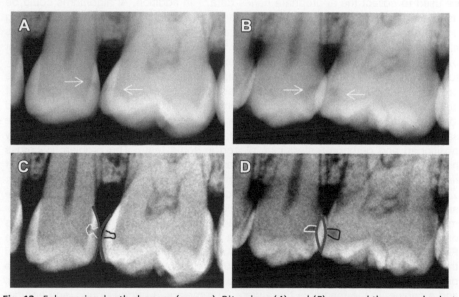

Fig. 12. False caries depth changes (*arrows*). Bitewings (*A*) and (*B*) exposed the same day but with about 15° change in horizontal beam projection. (*A*) #13D radiolucency just deeper than DEJ, #14M at DEJ. (*B*) False lesion depths #13D and #14M appear in outer one-third of the dentin. (*C*) Interproximal contact surfaces (*red*) no overlap. (*D*) Contact overlap (*red*).

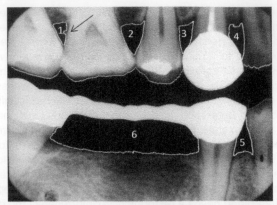

Fig. 13. Right bitewing radiograph automatically processed to identify interdental spaces (1–6). Computer able to identify interproximal surfaces for caries monitoring and alveolar bone crests for periodontal disease. Arrow in space 1 reveals calculus as an elevated loop on #3D surface. (*Courtesy of* British Institute of Radiology Publications, London; with permission.)

radiographic changes is judged by constancy of contact point overlap. The extra time and complexity for clinicians to perform these assessments makes this problem ideal for AI. What would a program have to do to automate the collection of the necessary radiographic information and integrate it with caries risk assessment? How can it provide a dentist with valid data to make an evidence-based decision to continue monitoring a lesion or apply topical fluoride and infiltrating resins or fluoride and restoration?

It has been proposed that iconic representations of the different lesion states could be used to collect the appropriate caries data.[20] In addition, AI algorithms could be used to integrate the clinical, radiographic, and caries risk into automatically generating a treatment plan at the whole body, oral cavity, and caries lesion levels. This has already been developed and demonstrated.[20] However, automating the measurement of radiolucency depth with contact point overlap validation is at least an order of magnitude increase in algorithm and programming complexity. To be clinically useful, the program must be able to take a bitewing radiograph recently created and compare it automatically with a similar earlier radiograph in the electronic chart. To do this it should identify a site; for example, #3 distal surface, in the current radiograph and find the same site in a previous one. Of course, the radiographs will not have been identically positioned and perhaps restorations placed in some teeth. The problem becomes how to find the same site in images that have changed. For a computer to do this, it has to create a list of what is in 1 bitewing and then find the same regions in the other.

One possible method is to find the interdental spaces (dark triangles) in an image and measure the width of the roots just below the crowns. Because molars and premolars have different widths, it is possible to classify a particular tooth as molar or as premolar and then by its position (maxilla or mandible) give it a tooth number. In **Fig. 13**, a bitewing radiograph has been automatically processed and the outline of the interdental spaces and interproximal surfaces shown. From this information, the program was able to create a list that in the maxilla there were 2 molars, 2 premolars, and a canine. In the mandible there were 2 premolars, a bridge pontic, and another tooth. More details of the computational theory and method have been published.[21,22]

The goals of this type of AI application would be to present a dentist with a report on the caries status of a sequential pair of bitewings; for example, "8/30/2017 #3D D1

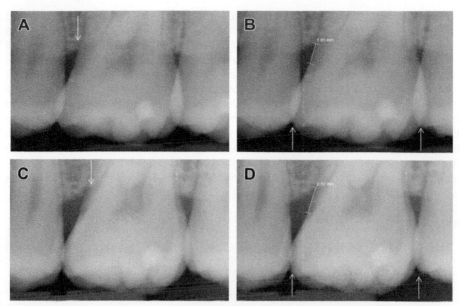

Fig. 14. Bitewing radiographs in A and C taken on the same day but with different horizontal X-ray beam directions. Interproximal surface overlap in A is greater than in C. The alveolar bone crest in C appears to be more apical than in A (*arrows*). The CEJ to crest distance is greater in D (2.32 mm) than B (1.85 mm) due solely to X-ray beam direction change. Changes in interproximal overlap (*arrows*) should alert an observer to this artifact.

deeper than 8/26/2016 #3 E2. However, overlap change. Caution advised as this is probably a false increase in depth".

The other major oral disease, periodontitis, can also suffer from image X-ray projection distortions leading to false bone changes. Similar to the checks for false caries changes, the alveolar bone crest to cementoenamel junction distance could be evaluated for changes in the vertical angulation of the X-ray beam for artifactual foreshortening or elongation in the distance measurements. Cuspal height variation between radiographs could reveal vertical angulation changes and contact point overlap changes indicate horizontal angulation variation. Both angular changes could produce errors in estimation of horizontal and vertical bone loss. In **Fig. 14** horizontal angulation changes have changed the size of a vertical defect on #14M.

In summary, current radiographic methods for estimating caries and periodontal lesion size and activity lack validation of false changes due to projection geometry alteration between serial radiographs. AI programs may provide a cost-effective solution to this problem.

SUMMARY

Digital imaging has fundamentally changed the way the dental office acquires, stores, and interacts with radiographic information. It has created exciting new opportunities to generate, enhance, and analyze radiographs. At the same time, it also has made the radiographic process much less intuitive. Numerous image processing and analysis tools are just a mouse click away, some of which have the power to radically change the way the radiographic information is perceived. The clinician is responsible for having a thorough understanding of the applications and limitations of these tools and the clinical implications of their use. Storing the raw data is always recommended to avoid permanent loss of important information and to be able to revert back to the original image. Findings noted on adjusted, filtered, or otherwise altered radiographs should be validated. Clinicians should also understand and test the limits of the operation of any filters they use. Any pathosis detected with the use of image enhancement tools should also be seen in the unenhanced image. The additional diagnostic power provided by image enhancement tools also carries a risk of misinterpretation and overdiagnosis that the clinician is responsible for understanding and avoiding. As the field continues to move forward, more advanced technologies will be introduced, including sophisticated analytical tools, new image reconstruction methods, and even AI. To maximize the health benefit to the patient, it is imperative that the dental professional is adequately trained in the use of these technologies and defers to specialists when appropriate.

REFERENCES

1. Shi XQ, Li G. Detection accuracy of approximal caries by black-and-white and color-coded digital radiographs. Oral Surg Oral Med Oral Pathol Oral Radiol Endod 2009;107(3):433–6.

2. Mol A, Yoon DC. Guide to digital radiographic imaging. J Calif Dent Assoc 2015; 43(9):503–11.

3. Schweitzer DM. A digital radiographic artifact: a clinical report. J Prosthet Dent 2010;103(6):326–9.

4. Tan TH. Uberschwinger artefact in computed radiographs. Br J Radiol 1997; 70(832):431.

5. Gormez O, Yilmaz HH. Image post-processing in dental practice. Eur J Dent 2009;3(4):343–7.

6. Webber RL, Ruttimann UE, Groenhuis RA. Computer correction of projective distortions in dental radiographs. J Dent Res 1984;63:1032–6.

7. Groenhuis RA, Webber RL, Ruttimann UE. Computerized tomosynthesis of dental tissues. Oral Surg Oral Med Oral Pathol 1983;56:206–14.

8. Ruttimann UE, Groenhuis RAJ, Webber RL. Computer tomosynthesis: a versatile 3-dimensional imaging technique. In Proc 7th Ann Symp on Computer Applications in medical care. New York, October 23–26, 1983.

9. Webber RL, Horton RA, Tyndall DA, et al. Tuned-aperture computed tomography (TACT™). Theory and application for three-dimensional dento-alveolar imaging. Dentomaxillofac Radiol 1997;26:53–62.

10. Shan J, Tucker AW, Gaalaas LR, et al. Stationary intra-oral digital tomosynthesis using a carbon nanotube X-ray source array. Dentomaxillofac Radiol 2015;44: 20150098.

11. McDavid WD, Welander U, Dove BS, et al. Digital imaging in rotational panoramic radiography. Dentomaxillofac Radiol 1995;24:68–75.

12. Barrett JF, Keat N. Artifacts in CT: recognition and avoidance. Radiographics 2004;24:1679–91.

13. Schulze R, Heil U, Gross D, et al. Artefacts in CBCT: a review. Dentomaxillofac Radiol 2011;40:265–73.

14. Morea C, Dominguez GC, Coutinho A, et al. Quantitative analysis of bone density in direct digital radiographs evaluated by means of computerized analysis of digital images. Dentomaxillofac Radiol 2010;39(6):356–61.

15. Stokholm R, Spin-Neto R, Nyengaard JR, et al. Comparison of radiographic and histological assessment of peri-implant bone around oral implants. Clin Oral Implants Res 2016;27:782–6.
16. Boden MA. Artificial intelligence and natural man. 2nd edition. MIT Press (MA): Basic Books; 1987.
17. Young DA, Nový BB, Zeller GG, et al. The American Dental Association caries classification system for clinical practice: a report of the American Dental Association Council on Scientific Affairs. J Am Dent Assoc 2015;146(2):79–86.
18. Ismail AI, Tellez M, Pitts NB, et al. Caries management pathways preserve dental tissues and promote oral health. Community Dent Oral Epidemiol 2013;41: e12–40.
19. Benn DK, Watson TF. Correlation between film position, bite-wing shadows, clinical pitfalls, and the histologic size of approximal lesions. Quintessence Int 1989;20(2):131–41.
20. Benn DK. Applying evidence-based dentistry to caries management in dental practice: a computerized approach. J Am Dent Assoc 2002;133(11):1543–8.
21. Benn DK. Automatic analysis of radiographic images: II. Software implementation and testing on bitewing radiographs. Dentomaxillofac Radiol 1991;20(4):193–9.
22. Benn DK. Automatic analysis of radiographic images: I. Theoretical considerations. Dentomaxillofac Radiol 1991;20(4):187–92.

Cone Beam Computed Tomography

Ibrahim Nasseh, DDS, DSO[a],*, Wisam Al-Rawi, DDS, MS[b]

KEYWORDS

- Computed tomography • Cone beam computed tomography • CBCT

KEY POINTS

- In the last several decades, the need for 3-dimensional images in dentistry have developed.
- While computed tomography (CT) allowed conditions to be diagnosed with 3D images, is is hospital-based, expensive, and exposes patients to relatively high doses of radiation.
- In the late 90's, a new technology using a cone-shaped beam, called the cone beam computerized tomography (CBCT), made the perception of 3D easy to dentists.
- Clinical needs, advantages, disadvantages, and indications for use of this imaging modality are described.

INTRODUCTION AND HISTORY

The development of computed tomography (CT) in 1972, which was reported in 1973,[1] enabled conditions to be diagnosed with 3-dimensional (3D) images. These devices were used in many fields, and their use in dentistry became more frequent with the advent of implant surgery. Although CT devices are becoming more compact, they continue to be relatively large, expensive, and expose patients to relatively high doses of radiation.

Arai and colleagues[2,3] set out to develop a compact CT apparatus specifically for use in dentistry. In 1997, they created a prototype-limited cone beam CT (CBCT) device for dental use that was dubbed Ortho-CT. In about 2 years after that achievement, the device was used in approximately 2000 cases to evaluate conditions, such as impacted teeth, apical lesions, and mandibular and maxillary diseases, both before and after surgery in the Department of Radiology at the Nihon University School of Dentistry Dental Hospital, proving highly successful.[4]

This prototype apparatus, the Ortho-CT, was an improved version of the Scanora (Soredex Corporation, Helsinki, Finland), a multifunctional pantomography imaging

[a] Department of Oral and Maxillofacial Radiology, Lebanese University, School of Dentistry, PO Box 166598, Beirut, Lebanon; [b] Private Practice, Horizon Dental, 742 Broadway, El Cajon, CA 92021, USA
* Corresponding author.
E-mail address: ibrahim.nasseh@gmail.com

Dent Clin N Am 62 (2018) 361–391
https://doi.org/10.1016/j.cden.2018.03.002
0011-8532/18/© 2018 Elsevier Inc. All rights reserved.

dental.theclinics.com

apparatus. In the Ortho-CT, the section where the film cassette was installed was replaced with an image intensifier, resulting in improved operability, resolution, and reduced radiation doses.[2,3]

In 2000, this technology was transferred to Morita Co Ltd through the Nihon University Business Incubation Center. The 3DX multi-image micro-CT was developed as a limited CBCT device for practical use, enabling 3D imaging of the hard tissues (ie, bone, tooth) of the maxillofacial, ear, and nose regions.[5]

The NewTom QR 9000 (Mozzo and colleagues)[6], a volume imaging machine produced in Italy, received FDA (Food and Drug Administration) approval in April 2001 and then CDA (Canadian Dental Association) approval in August 2002.

The NewTom QR 9000 has been designed specifically to image the maxillofacial region. In a single scan, the x-ray source and a reciprocating x-ray sensor rotate around the head and acquire 360 pictures (one image per degree of rotation) using 17 seconds of accumulated exposure time.

CONE BEAM COMPUTED TOMOGRAPHY FUNDAMENTALS

CBCT uses an extraoral imaging scanner, specifically designed for head and neck imaging that produces 3D scans of the maxillofacial skeleton. It involves a unit that can be comparable in size with a conventional panoramic radiographic machine.

Cone beam machines use x-rays in the form of a large cone covering the head surface to be examined; instead of a linear array of detectors as in CT, a 2-dimensional (2D) planar detector is used.

Because the cone beam irradiates a large volume area instead of a thin slice, the machine does not need to rotate as many times as CT, it rotates once giving all the information necessary to reconstruct the region of interest (ROI).

This technique allows clinicians to obtain 2D reconstructed images in all planes, and reconstructions in 3 dimensions with low level exposure to x-radiation.[7]

Supine Versus Seated Positioning

There are many types of CBCT machines with different characteristics. One of these differences is the position of patients in the machine: standing, sitting, or lying on a table.

Clinicians are used to sitting or standing positioning for in-office 2D imaging. For 3D cone beam imaging, minimizing patient motion is critical for high-quality results to reduce blur and motion artifacts.[8]

Image Intensifier Versus Flat Panel Efficiency over Time

In early generation CBCT systems, image intensifiers were commonly used. Currently, different types of flat panel detectors (FPDs) are used instead, as these detectors are distortion free, have a higher dose efficiency and a wider dynamic range, and can be produced with either a smaller or larger field of view (FOV). Most existing CBCT systems use indirect FPDs whereby a layer of scintillator material, either gadolinium oxysulfide or cesium iodide, is used to convert x-ray photons to light photons, which in turn are converted into electrical signals.[9–11]

Field of View

The size of the FOV describes the scan volume of a particular CBCT machine and depends on the detector's size and shape, the beam projection geometry, and the ability to collimate the beam, which differs from one manufacturer to another. Beam collimation limits the patients' ionizing radiation exposure to the ROI and ensures that an appropriate FOV can be selected based on the specific case.

In general, CBCT units can be classified into small, medium, and large volume based on the size of their FOV (**Fig. 1**). Small-volume CBCT machines are used to scan a range from a sextant or a quadrant to one jaw only. They generally offer higher image resolution because x-ray scattering (noise) is reduced as the FOV decreases. Medium-volume CBCT machines are used to scan both jaws, whereas large FOV machines allow the visualization of the entire head commonly used in orthodontic and orthognathic surgery treatment planning. The main limitation of large FOV CBCT units is the size of the field irradiated. Unless the smallest voxel size is selected in the larger FOV machines, there is also a reduction in image resolution as compared with intraoral radiographs or small FOV CBCT machines with inherent small voxel sizes.

Limiting the scan volume should be based on the clinician's judgment for the situation. For most dental implant applications, a small or medium FOV is sufficient to visualize the ROI. Small-volume CBCT machines are more popular in endodontic cases because they provide the following advantages over larger-volume CBCT:

Increased spatial resolution
Decreased radiation exposure to patients
Smaller volume to be interpreted
Less expensive machines

Cone Beam Computed Tomography Image Formation

The image formation process consists of 2 major stages: *acquisition* and *reconstruction, followed by image display*.[8,9] To facilitate data handling, some machines require that data are acquired by a separate acquisition computer and transferred to another processing computer (workstation) for reconstruction. Cone beam data reconstruction is usually performed on Windows-based platforms.

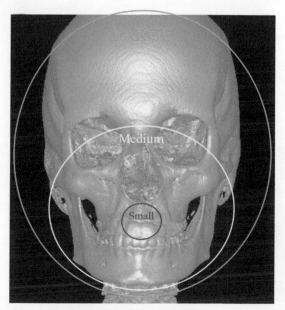

Fig. 1. Area covered by small, medium, and large FOVs.

Acquisition stage

Cone beam acquisition techniques mostly use a single 180° rotation or more in which the x-ray source and a reciprocating x-ray detector are attached by an arm and they rotate around patients' heads.

The FOV determined by the area of interest depends primarily on the detector's size, beam projection geometry, and selected collimation whenever available.

The primary images captured during a CBCT scan consist of a sequence of 2D projection images: projection data, raw data, basis projections, or basis frames.

Projection data are promptly reconstructed into what constitutes the real outcome of CBCT: a volumetric data set (**Fig. 2**).

The number of projection images comprising the data set varies depending on the system; this number is determined both by the frame rate and the exposure cycle.

The higher the frame rate, the more information that is available to construct the image; a higher frame rate with frame averaging and a slightly lower signal can still achieve a better signal-to-noise ratio (SNR) than a lower frame rate.

$$\text{Signal to} - \text{noise ratio (SNR)} = \frac{\text{mean signal value}}{\text{standard deviation}} = \frac{\text{useful image information}}{\text{random information}}$$

Zhao and colleagues[12] revealed a nonmonotonic relationship between image noise and the number of projections (Nproj) at a fixed total dose: noise decreased with increasing Nproj because of a reduction of view sampling effects in the regime Nproj of 200 or less, greater than which noise increased with Nproj due to increased electronic noise.

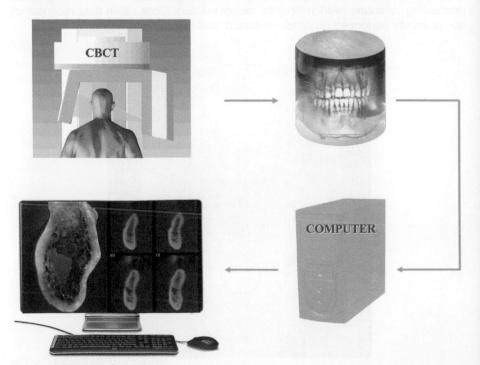

Fig. 2. CBCT image formation.

Several units have variable frame rates. Rotation times range between 10 and 40 seconds, so the exposure time is comparable with that for a standard panoramic image.

On CBCT units that have a pulse generator, the number of projection images obtained correlates to the radiation exposure to patients.

In some cases, multiple consecutive scans are acquired, which are then merged (ie, stitched) into one image. This merger can be carried out to combine 2 or more small-diameter FOVs (**Fig. 3**) or 2 small-height FOVs. Between the scans, the chair or C-arm moves along a preset path, leaving a small overlap between the images. Stitching of the image volume could be carried out through a simple overlap (as the relative movement of patients between the scans is known exactly) or through automatic matching of the images using image registration.[13]

Artifact Reduction

An image artifact is a visualized structure in the reconstructed data that is not present in the object under investigation. Artifacts can significantly affect the quality of CBCT images by decreasing the contrast between adjacent objects and ultimately lead to an inaccurate or false diagnosis.[14]

Among different kinds of artifacts (such as scatter, noise artifacts, and others), beam-hardening artifacts are considered to be the most prominent artifacts induced by dental implants and metallic restorations.[15] By definition, beam hardening is the process by which low-energy photons in a polychromatic beam

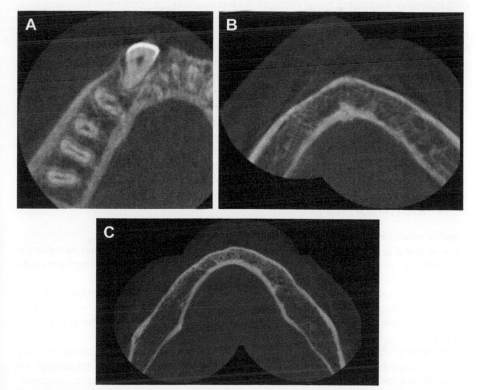

Fig. 3. Image stitching in CBCT. (*A*) Small FOV covering the right mandible. (*B*) Stitching of 2 FOVs. (*C*) Stitching of 3 FOVs, covering a larger area of the mandible.

are attenuated after passing through metallic objects, such as dental implants, leading to an increase in beam average energy level, that is, the beam becomes harder.

The sensor records too much energy because only the higher-energy rays penetrate the implant, whereas the lower-energy rays of the polychromatic spectrum emitted by the x-ray source will suffer substantial absorption when passing through dense objects. Hence, the intensity recorded will be too high (ie, the gray value too dark) in relation to other less-dense structures.[15]

Beam-hardening artifact in dental implants will appear clinically as dark bands or a halo around an implant or as an erroneous dark hourglasslike shape in between implants. This artifact will change visibility and accuracy of the surrounding peri-implant bone interphase, leading to inaccurate assessment of the peri-implant region.

Metal Artifact Reduction Methods

Metal artifact reduction can be carried out by[16]

1. Adaptive scanning technique
2. Specific reconstruction algorithm (preprocessing technique)
3. Postprocessing technique

Adaptive scanning technique

FOV, kilovoltage peak, milliampere, and voxel size are the effective parameters in decreasing or increasing metal artifacts during scanning procedure.[16,17]

Selection of FOV and voxel size can impact diagnosing dental peri-implant defects. It is possible to obtain smaller voxel sizes with smaller FOVs, leading to improvement in spatial resolution of high-contrast structures. Decreasing voxel size, a better spatial resolution image can be obtained but at the expense of a greater the noise.[18]

A more pronounced beam hardening effect was observed in machines working at 80 kV and less artifact in machines with a higher kilovoltage range (120–140 kV).[15,16]

This finding is explained by the fact that increasing the tube voltage increases the effective x-ray energy, which can improve beam penetration and, thus, reduce the missing projection data, in turn reducing the artifact areas.[19]

Although it can be expected that many projections leads to artifact reduction, there was no perceptible difference between high-milliampere and low-milliampere protocols.[16] This finding means that increasing the milliampere will only lead to minor improvements in image quality.

Specific reconstruction algorithms (preprocessing technique)

Several metal artifact reducing methods for the CBCT system have been proposed in the past few years, most of which need to prereconstruct FOV and segment metal areas in the 3D space.[20]

In preprocessing algorithm, the metal part in the basis projection is first identified and then, using the interpolation algorithm, metal projection data are modified. From these preprocessed raw data, images are reconstructed and metal section is retrieved.[21]

Nowadays, CBCT manufacturing companies are actively developing artifact-reducing algorithms to be used during image reconstruction. These processes are rather time consuming and may further slow down the total reconstruction process.

Because these artifacts are inherent to the data acquisition process, they cannot be avoided completely.

Postprocessing technique

This technique applies the metal artifact reduction algorithm on Digital Imaging and Communications in Medicine files, not on raw projection data; this means that postprocessing is based on segmentation and modification of metal areas in each projection image and reconstruction of the final image with modified data.

In terms of artifact reduction, preprocessing of the actual physical image acquisition is superior to postprocessing of affected data.[21]

Reconstruction After transfer to the workstation computer, the basis images are processed, which includes correction of the images both visually and geometrically and final application of a reconstruction algorithm.

Once all slices have been reconstructed, they can be recombined into a single volume for visualization.

Reconstruction times vary depending on the acquisition parameters (voxel size, FOV, Nproj), hardware (processing speed, data throughput from the acquisition computer to the workstation), and software (reconstruction algorithms) used.

Reconstruction should be accomplished in an acceptable time (less than 5 minutes) to complement patient flow.

Image display and manipulation The main functions are

- Multiplanar reformatting (MPR) (**Fig. 4**)
- Panoramic or curvilinear (**Fig. 5**) and cross-sectional reconstructions (**Fig. 6**)
- Maximum intensity projection (MIP) and volume rendering (**Fig. 7**)

Advantages of Cone Beam Computed Tomography Scanners over Medical Computed Tomography Scanners

- The cost of equipment is approximately 3 to 5 times less than traditional medical CT.
- The equipment is substantially lighter and smaller.
- CBCT has a better spatial resolution (ie, smaller pixels).
- No special electrical requirements are needed.
- No floor strengthening is required.
- The room does not need to be cooled.
- It is very easy to operate and to maintain; little technician training is required.

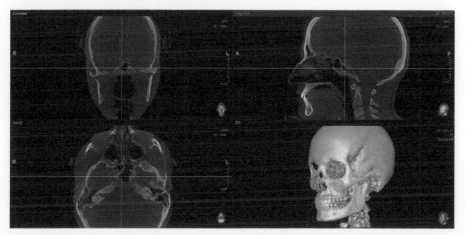

Fig. 4. MPR screen, with the coronal, sagittal, axial, and 3D rendering views.

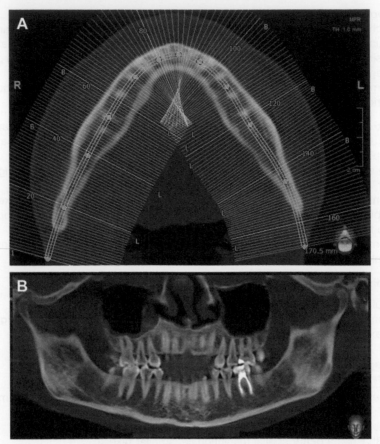

Fig. 5. Panoramic image reconstruction (*A*) along a curve drawn by the user in the axial plane (*B*).

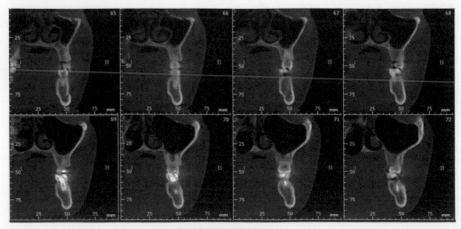

Fig. 6. Upper and lower cross-sectional reconstructions.

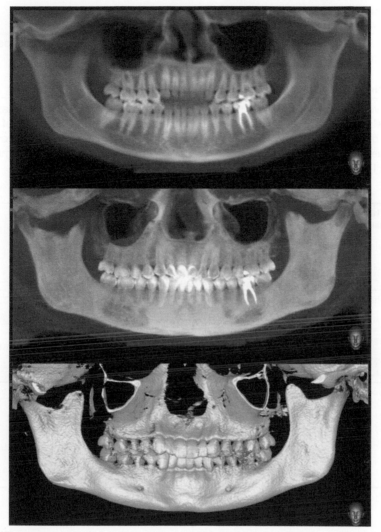

Fig. 7. Panoramic reconstruction (*upper*), transformed with an MIP (*middle*), and volume rendering (*lower*).

- Some CBCT manufacturers and vendors are dedicated to the dental market, which makes for a greater appreciation of dentists' needs.
- In most CBCT machines, patients are seated, as compared with lying down in a medical CT unit. This upright position, together with the open design of CBCT, results in almost complete elimination of claustrophobia and greatly enhances patient comfort and acceptance. The upright position is also thought by many to provide a more realistic picture of condylar positions during a temporomandibular joint (TMJ) examination.
- It is a cost-effective tool for imaging a wide range of clinical problems.
- Both jaws can be imaged at the same time (depending on the specifications of the machine).
- The radiation dose is considerably less than a medical CT.

Limitation of Cone Beam Computed Tomography Compared with Medical Computed Tomography Scanners

- There is lower contrast resolution, which means less discrimination between different tissue types (ie, bone, teeth, and soft tissue).[22]

Applications in Dentistry

The advent of CBCT has made it possible to visualize the dentition, the maxillofacial skeleton, and the relationship of anatomic structures in 3D. The use of CBCT in the dental profession is increasing exponentially because of an increase of equipment manufacturers and the growing acceptance of this imaging modality (**Table 1**).

Table 1
Summary of applications cone beam computed tomography in dentistry

1. Implants planning	1. Presence of some kind of pathology 2. Location of anatomic features 3. Location of osseous morphology 4. Amount of bone available
2. Orthodontics	1. Assessment of palatal bone thickness 2. Skeletal growth pattern 3. Severity of tooth impaction 4. Arch expansion 5. Position of the mandibular condyles 6. Airway analysis 7. Orthognathic surgery
3. Endodontics	1. Evaluation of root canal morphology 2. 3D representation of periapical pathology 3. Assessment of pathosis of endodontic and nonendodontic origin 4. Identifying an untreated or missed canal 5. Visualizing overextended root canal obturation material 6. Analysis of external and internal root resorption 7. Evaluation of vertical and horizontal root fractures
4. Pathology	1. Developmental abnormalities 2. Cystic and benign tumors 3. Reactive lesions 4. Inflammatory lesions 5. Malignancy
5. Maxillary sinus	1. Dento-apical pathology of the maxillary posterior teeth 2. Soft tissue thickening of the sinus floor mucosa 3. Assessment of vertical bone height before placement of implants 4. Assessment of bone graft
6. Trauma and surgery	1. Trauma 2. Follow-up
7. TMJ	1. Condylar head shape and position 2. Erosion and osteoarthritic changes
8. Periodontics	1. Assessment of bone loss 2. Evaluation of bony defects 3. Preperiodontal and postperiodontal surgery assessment 4. Bone graft evaluation
9. Airways	1. Assessment of total airway space volume 2. Soft tissue changes

Implant planning

Endosseous dental implants were introduced following the discovery of osseointegration by Dr P. Brånemark.[23] He made this discovery accidentally in 1952 when he was studying blood flow in rabbit femurs by placing titanium chambers in their bone; over time the chamber became firmly affixed to the bone and could not be removed.[23,24]

In 1978, Brånemark presented a 2-stage threaded titanium root-form implant; he developed and tested a system using pure titanium screws, which he termed *fixtures*. These fixtures were first placed in his patients in 1965 and were the first to be well documented and the most well-maintained dental implants thus far. With his implant came the concept of osseointegration.[24] Dental implants have now become a widely used treatment option for replacement of lost teeth.

The success of dental implant restorations depends, in part, on adequate diagnostic information about bony structures of the oral region. Acquiring this information usually requires some form of imaging, which may vary from simple 2D views, such as panoramic radiographs, to more complex views in multiple planes, depending on the case and the experience of the practitioner.

The objective of preoperative dental implant imaging is to gain the following infor mation about the potential implant site:

1. Presence of some kind of pathologic conditions (**Figs. 8** and **9**)
2. Location of anatomic features that should be avoided when placing an implant, such as the maxillary sinus, nasopalatine canal, inferior alveolar canal, and the mental canal and foramen (see **Fig. 9**)
3. Location of osseous morphology, including knife-edge ridges, location and depth of the submandibular fossa, developmental variations, postextraction irregularities, enlarged marrow spaces, cortical integrity and thickness, and trabecular bone density
4. Amount of bone available for implant placement (**Fig. 10**)[25]

The American Academy of Oral and Maxillofacial Radiology (AAOMR) recommends panoramic and orthogonal cross-sectional imaging for all implant site evaluations and endorses conventional tomography as the most cost-effective and lowest-radiation-risk modality available today for most patients. The AAOMR also recommends that the execution of imaging and interpretation of the resultant images not be attempted without adequate training and that, before restoration or placement of an implant, the clinician seeks such training or obtains the needed radiographic information from qualified experts.[25]

Lastly, the AAOMR published a position article for the use of radiology in dental implantology with emphasis on the use of CBCT.[26] The recommendations are presented in **Table 2**.

Orthodontics

CBCT technology has made an impact on current practices in orthodontics, influencing the clinical application of orthodontics. Many orthodontic conditions cannot be appraised adequately by using conventional radiographs. For example, assessment of palatal bone thickness, skeletal growth pattern, severity of tooth impaction, arch expansion, nonextraction treatments, and so forth cannot be determined completely without 3D imaging. In addition, the position of the mandibular condyles in the glenoid fossa and the association of airway abnormalities to craniofacial morphology cannot be evaluated using conventional imaging approaches.[27–32]

The use of CBCT in orthognathic surgery (**Fig. 11**) is becoming paramount.[33]

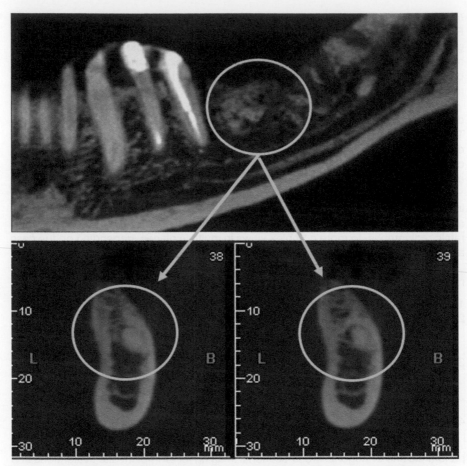

Fig. 8. A high-density region at the future implant site on the reconstructed panoramic; cross sections reveal a residual tooth structure (*lower circles*).

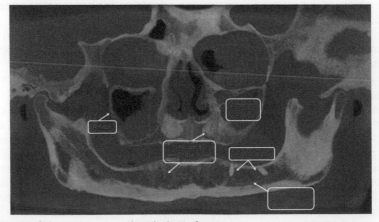

Fig. 9. Some of the anatomic and pathologic features.

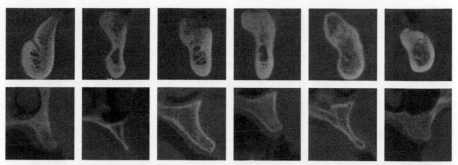

Fig. 10. The unlimited possibilities of nature concerning morphology, developmental variations, degree of resorption, and so forth.

Table 2
Summary of the position statement of the American Academy of Oral and Maxillofacial Radiology on selection criteria for the use of radiology in dental implantology with emphasis on cone beam computed tomography

Recommendation 1	Panoramic radiography should be used as the imaging modality of choice in the initial evaluation of dental implant patients.
Recommendation 2	Use intraoral periapical radiography to supplement the preliminary information from panoramic radiography.
Recommendation 3	Do not use cross-sectional imaging, including CBCT, as an initial diagnostic imaging examination.
Recommendation 4	The radiographic examination of any potential implant site should include cross-sectional imaging orthogonal to the site of interest.
Recommendation 5	CBCT should be considered as the imaging modality of choice for preoperative cross-sectional imaging of potential implant sites.
Recommendation 6	CBCT should be considered when clinical conditions indicate a need for augmentation procedures or site development before the placement of dental implants: (1) sinus augmentation, (2) block or particulate bone grafting, (3) ramus or symphysis grafting, (4) assessment of impacted teeth, (5) evaluation of bone volume.
Recommendation 7	CBCT imaging should be considered if bone reconstruction and augmentation procedures (for example, ridge preservation or bone grafting) have been performed to treat bone volume deficiencies before implant placement.
Recommendation 8	In the absence of clinical signs or symptoms, use intraoral periapical radiography for the postoperative assessment of implants. Panoramic radiographs may be indicated for more extensive implant therapy cases.
Recommendation 9	Use cross-sectional imaging (particularly CBCT) immediately postoperatively, only if patients present with implant mobility or altered sensation, especially if the fixture is in the posterior mandible.
Recommendation 10	Do not use CBCT imaging for the periodic review of clinically asymptomatic implants.
Recommendation 11	Cross-sectional imaging, optimally CBCT, should be considered if implant retrieval is anticipated.

Data from Tyndall DA, Price JB, Tetradis S, et al. Position statement of the American Academy of Oral and Maxillofacial Radiology on selection criteria for the use of radiology in dental implantology with emphasis on cone beam computed tomography. Oral Surg Oral Med Oral Pathol Oral Radiol 2012;113(6):817–26.

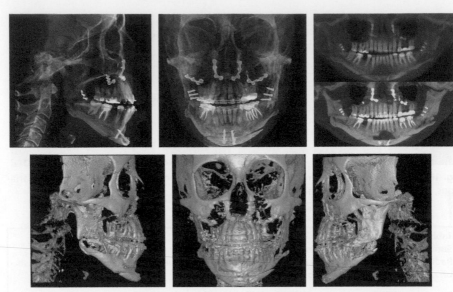

Fig. 11. Three-dimensional multiple reconstructions after orthognathic surgery.

Some investigators[34] are using CBCT-synthesized images for orthodontic tracing, measurements, and planning (**Fig. 12**). They find that a synthesized cephalometric image can be used to delineate ambiguous visual landmarks, such as porion, and avoid measurement inaccuracy found on conventional cephalogram. Although this practice

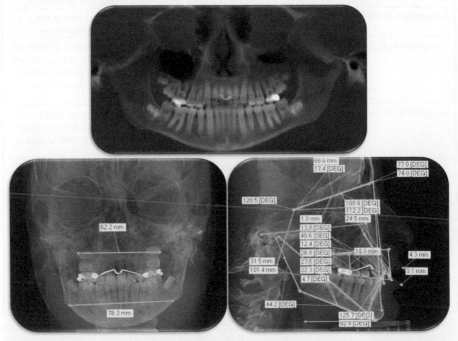

Fig. 12. Example of synthesized panoramic and cephalograms, with orthodontics drawing of points and planes.

is becoming popular, further studies are needed to determine when it should be ordered for orthodontic cases, especially because most patients are young and the radiation dose associated with CBCT is higher than the traditional plain radiograph.[22]

Imaging selection recommendations, optimization protocols, and radiation-dose risk-assessment strategies were developed to assist professional clinical judgment on the use of CBCT in orthodontics. The following position statement and guidelines were developed by board-certified orthodontists and oral and maxillofacial radiologists convened by the AAOMR.[35]

A summary of this position statement is presented in **Table 3**.

Endodontics

Conventional 2D periapical radiographs still play a predominant role in the evaluation of periapical pathosis in today's endodontic field because they provide clinicians with cost-effective and high-resolution imaging. Perhaps the most important advantage of CBCT in endodontics is that it demonstrates anatomic features in 3D that intraoral, panoramic, and cephalometric images cannot.[36,37]

Indications of CBCT in endodontics include

- Evaluation of root canal morphology (**Fig. 13**; best way is to look at axial slices, from the crown to the root)
- 3D representation of periapical pathology (**Fig. 14**)
- Assessment of pathosis of endodontic and nonendodontic origin (**Fig. 15**)
- Identifying an untreated or missed canal (**Fig. 16**)
- Visualizing overextended root canal obturation material (**Fig. 17**)
- Analysis of external and internal root resorption (**Fig. 18**)
- Evaluation of vertical and horizontal root fractures (**Fig. 19**)

The American Association of Endodontists and the AAOMR published the following updated joint position statement intended to provide scientifically based guidance to clinicians regarding the use of CBCT in endodontic treatment[38,39] (**Table 4**).

Pathology

If a clinician detects or is suspicious of an abnormality or a lesion on 2D radiographs, such as periapical and panoramic, CBCT can be used to further assess the ROI in cross sections[40] (**Fig. 20**). Using cross sections from a CBCT scan, with absence of magnification and superimposition of structures, allows the clinician to confirm or rule out suspected pathosis.

Pathology, particularly bone, teeth, and airway spaces, can be detected on CBCT, thanks to good contrast of hard tissue structures. When compared with a medical CT scan, soft tissue contrast on CBCT is poor because of lower SNR caused by scattering radiation from larger projection image dimensions and lower mA settings.

High bone contrast allows visualization of lesions affecting bone, including developmental abnormalities, cystic and benign tumors, reactive lesions, malignancy, and inflammatory lesions[28] (**Fig. 21**).

Studies have shown that CBCT examinations enable the surgeon to produce a more conservative treatment approach, which reduces iatrogenic damages and is more acceptable to patients.[41]

Maxillary sinus

CBCT is used for the evaluation of the paranasal sinuses, mainly the maxillary sinus because of its close relationship to the maxillary posterior teeth. Pathology around the apices of the maxillary posterior teeth can show up around the sinus floor. The maxillary sinus appears fundamentally radiolucent (low density) because it is an

Table 3
Summary of the position statement and guidelines of the American Academy of Oral and Maxillofacial Radiology and Orthodontists

1. Image appropriately according to clinical condition.	*Recommendation 1.1.* The decision to perform a CBCT examination is based on patients' history, clinical examination, available radiographic imaging, and the presence of a clinical condition for which the benefits to the diagnosis and/or treatment plan outweigh the potential risks of exposure to radiation, especially in the case of a child or young adult. *Recommendation 1.2.* Use CBCT when the clinical question for which imaging is required cannot be answered adequately by lower-dose conventional dental radiography or alternate nonionizing imaging modalities. *Recommendation 1.3.* Avoid using CBCT on patients to obtain data that can be provided by alternate nonionizing modalities (eg, to produce virtual orthodontic study models). *Recommendation 1.4.* Use a CBCT protocol that restricts the FOV, minimizes exposure (milliampere and kilovoltage peak), the number of basis images, and resolution yet permits adequate visualization of the region of interest. *Recommendation 1.5.* Avoid taking a CBCT scan solely to produce a lateral cephalogram and/or panoramic view if the CBCT would result in higher radiation exposure than would conventional imaging. *Recommendation 1.6.* Avoid taking conventional 2D radiographs if the clinical examination indicates that a CBCT study is indicated for proper diagnosis and/or treatment planning or if a recent CBCT study is available.
2. Assess the radiation dose risk.	*Recommendation 2.1.* Consider the RRL when assessing the imaging risk for imaging procedures over a course of orthodontic treatment. *Recommendation 2.2.* Because CBCT exposes patients to ionizing radiation that may pose elevated risks to some patients (pregnant or younger patients), explain and disclosure to patient's radiation exposure risks, benefits and imaging modality alternatives and document this in the patients' records.
3. Minimize patient radiation exposure.	*Recommendation 3.1.* Perform CBCT imaging with acquisition parameters adjusted to the nominal settings consistent with providing appropriate images of task specific diagnostic quality for the desired diagnostic information required. *Recommendation 3.2.* When other factors remain the same, reduce the size of the FOV to match the ROI; however, selection of FOV may result in automatic or default changes in other technical factors (eg, milliampere) that should be considered because these concomitant changes can result in an increase in dose. *Recommendation 3.3.* Use patient protective shielding (such as lead torso aprons and consider the use of thyroid shields) when possible (eg, maxillary only scan) to minimize exposure to radiosensitive organs outside the FOV of the exposure. *Recommendation 3.4.* Ensure that all CBCT equipment is properly installed, routinely calibrated and updated, and meets all governmental requirements and regulations.

(continued on next page)

Table 3 (continued)	
4. Maintain professional competency in performing and interpreting CBCT studies.	*Recommendation 4.1.* Clinicians have an obligation to attain and improve their professional skills through lifelong learning in regards to performing CBCT examinations as well as interpreting the resultant images. Clinicians need to attend continuing education courses to maintain familiarity with the technical and operational aspects of CBCT and to maintain current knowledge of scientific advances and health risks associated with the use of CBCT. *Recommendation 4.2.* Clinicians have legal responsibilities when operating CBCT equipment and interpreting images and are expected to comply with all governmental and third party payer (eg, Medicare) regulations. *Recommendation 4.3.* It is important that patients/guardians know about the limitations of CBCT with regard to visualization of soft tissues, artifacts and noise.

Data from American Academy of Oral and Maxillofacial Radiology. Clinical recommendations regarding use of cone beam computed tomography in orthodontics [corrected]. Position statement by the American Academy of Oral and Maxillofacial Radiology. Oral Surg Oral Med Oral Pathol Oral Radiol 2013;116(2):238-57.

air-filled cavity. Any alteration in the sinus, including soft tissue thickening of the sinus floor mucosa or soft tissue growth in the sinus, can show up as a radiopaque (high density) entity[42] (**Fig. 22**).

CBCT is also useful for the assessment of vertical bone height before the placement of implants and assessment of bone graft in maxillary sinus-lift procedures (**Fig. 23**).

Trauma and surgery

Maxillofacial and jaw fractures due to trauma from motor vehicle accidents, assaults, and accidents can be evaluated using CBCT.[43] Medical CT is usually the modality of choice, as patients are brought to the emergency department at the hospital first and medical CT provides better soft tissue and hard tissue evaluation. CBCT can be useful for follow-up after surgery[44,45] (**Fig. 24**).

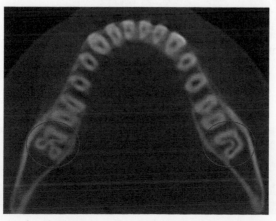

Fig. 13. Visualization of molars' root canal morphology on the axial view (*circles*).

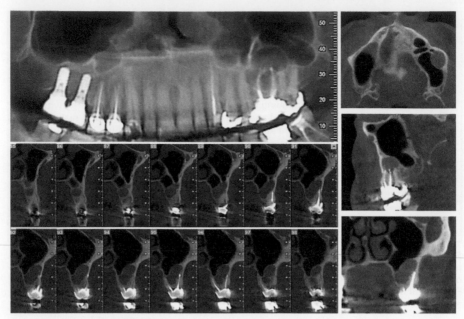

Fig. 14. A 3D representation of a periapical pathology.

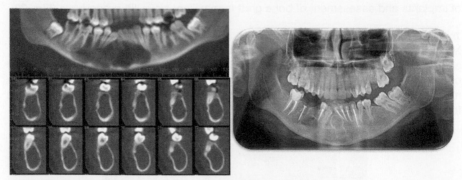

Fig. 15. Assessment of a pathosis of nonendodontic origin.

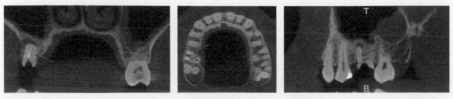

Fig. 16. The arrows point to an untreated canal in the 3 planes.

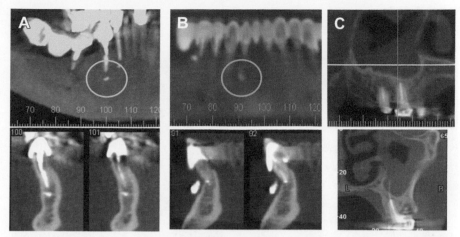

Fig. 17. Overextended root canal obturation material on the panoramic reconstruction (*circle*). Their corresponding on the cross-sections (*A*) In the bone; (*B*) outside the bone; (*C*) in the sinus.

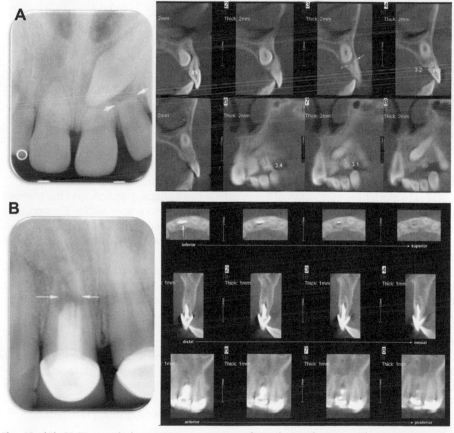

Fig. 18. (*A*) CBCT revealed extensive resorption of tooth number 10 with an average of 3 mm of root structure remaining (*arrowheads*). Tooth number 9 seems to be unaffected. (*B*) The central incisor shows internal root resorption (*arrows*). External root resorption may be present apically, although this may represent a sequela of the internal resorption. On the cross sections, the internal resorption extends from the apex into the postspace. A low density image is present superior and distal to the apex of central incisor and seems to communicate with the apex.

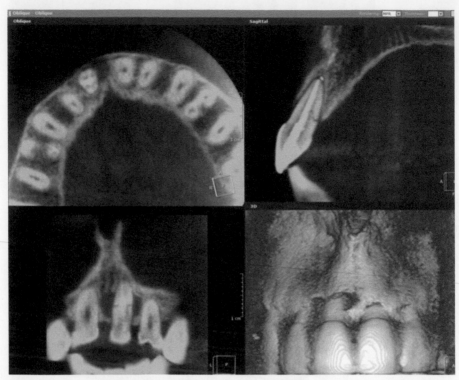

Fig. 19. Fractured central as appearing in 3D views.

Temporomandibular joint

CBCT is useful for the evaluation of the condylar head shape, position, and the glenoid fossa. It has a lower radiation dose than CT, and it is more accessible. Erosion and osteoarthritic changes can be detected (**Fig. 25**). Current CBCT software allows a specialized view for TMJ where cross sections are generated along the condylar head anteroposteriorly and mediolaterally.[46,47]

Because of the poor soft tissue contrast of CBCT, it cannot detect changes in the articular disc, such as disc displacement and derangement. MRI remains the gold standard for the evaluation of the disc's position and other soft tissue components of TMJ.[48,49]

Periodontics

CBCT can be used for accurate assessment of bone loss and 3D evaluation of bony defects due to periodontal diseases (**Fig. 26**). In addition, preperiodontal and postperiodontal surgery assessment can be carried out to evaluate whether there is progress of the condition or if the case is stable. CBCT is used for post bone graft evaluation to check the dimensions of the graft and whether further bone grafting is needed.[50–53]

Airways

Airway spaces commonly visualized in maxillofacial CBCT include nasopharyngeal and oropharyngeal airways. CBCT is used for the assessment of total airway space volume. Constriction or reduction in airway space area or volume can possibly indicate the presence of a sleep apnea.

Table 4
Summary of the updated joint position statement of the American Association of Endodontists and the American Academy of Oral and Maxillofacial Radiology

Recommendation 1	Intraoral radiographs should be considered the imaging modality of choice in the evaluation of endodontic patients.
Recommendation 2	Limited FOV CBCT should be considered the imaging modality of choice for diagnosis in patients who present with contradictory or nonspecific clinical signs and symptoms associated with untreated or previously endodontically treated teeth.
Recommendation 3	Limited FOV CBCT should be considered the imaging modality of choice for initial treatment of teeth with the potential for extra canals and suspected complex morphology, such as mandibular anterior teeth, maxillary and mandibular premolars and molars, and dental anomalies.
Recommendation 4	If a preoperative CBCT has not been taken, limited FOV CBCT should be considered as the imaging modality of choice for intra-appointment identification and localization of calcified canals.
Recommendation 5	Intraoral radiographs should be considered the imaging modality of choice for immediate postoperative imaging.
Recommendation 6	Limited FOV CBCT should be considered the imaging modality of choice if clinical examination and 2D intraoral radiography are inconclusive in the detection of vertical root fracture.
Recommendation 7	Limited FOV CBCT should be the imaging modality of choice when evaluating the nonhealing of previous endodontic treatment to help determine the need for further treatment, such as nonsurgical, surgical, or extraction.
Recommendation 8	Limited FOV CBCT should be the imaging modality of choice for nonsurgical retreatment to assess endodontic treatment complications, such as overextended root canal obturation material, separated endodontic instruments, and localization of perforations.
Recommendation 9	Limited FOV CBCT should be considered as the imaging modality of choice for presurgical treatment planning to localize root apex/apices and to evaluate the proximity to adjacent anatomic structures.
Recommendation 10	Limited FOV CBCT should be considered as the imaging modality of choice for surgical placement of implants.
Recommendation 11	Limited FOV CBCT should be considered the imaging modality of choice for diagnosis and management of limited dentoalveolar trauma, root fractures, luxation, and/or displacement of teeth and localized alveolar fractures, in the absence of other maxillofacial or soft tissue injury that may require other advanced imaging modalities.
Recommendation 12	Limited FOV CBCT is the imaging modality of choice in the localization and differentiation of external and internal resorptive defects and the determination of appropriate treatment and prognosis.
Recommendation 13	In the absence of clinical signs or symptoms, intraoral radiographs should be considered the imaging modality of choice for the evaluation of healing following nonsurgical and surgical endodontic treatment.
Recommendation 14	In the absence of signs and symptoms, if limited FOV CBCT was the imaging modality of choice at the time of evaluation and treatment, it may be the modality of choice for follow-up evaluation. In the presence of signs and symptoms, refer to recommendation 7.

Data from Fayad MI, Nair M, Levin MD, et al, Special Committee to Revise the Joint AAE/AAOMR Position Statement on Use of CBCT in Endodontics. AAE and AAOMR joint position statement: use of cone beam computed tomography in endodontics 2015 update. Oral Surg Oral Med Oral Pathol Oral Radiol 2015;120(4):508–12.

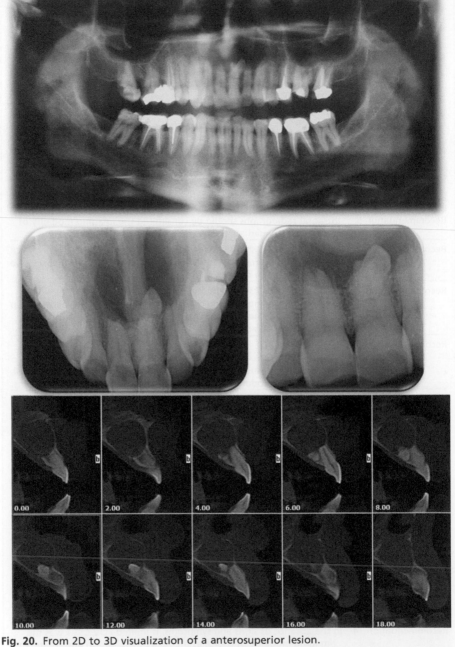

Fig. 20. From 2D to 3D visualization of a anterosuperior lesion.

CBCT can be useful in sleep studies. CBCT devices that have patients lying in the supine position while being scanned are better suited for airway studies, as patients are positioned in a similar fashion to a sleeping position; thus, soft tissue changes due to gravity can be better assessed (**Fig. 27**).

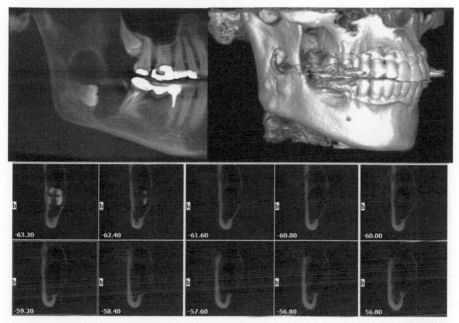

Fig. 21. Panoramic, 3D rendering, and cross-sectional views of an extended low-density image with tooth involvement.

Some CBCT imaging software provides specific tools to allow clinicians to accurately assess the airway space automatically, semiautomatically, or manually.[54,55]

However, the accuracy of these measurements can vary; more scientific studies are needed to confirm their validity.

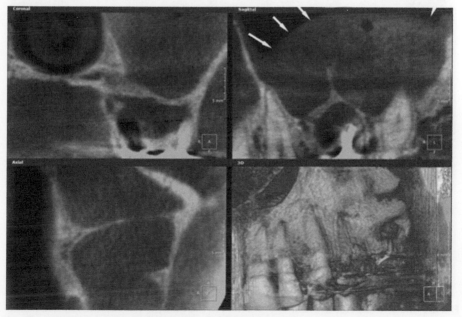

Fig. 22. Arrows point to sinusitis within the maxillary sinus.

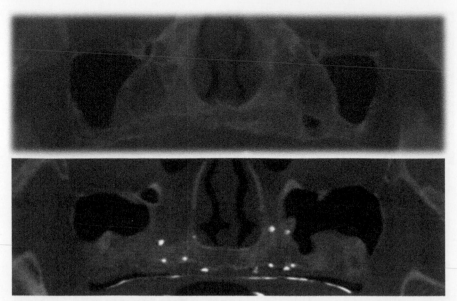

Fig. 23. Panoramic reconstruction of the maxillary sinus before and after bone grafting procedures.

Ethical and legal

According to American Dental Association Council on Scientific Affairs[56] and AAOMR,[26] clinicians who acquire dental radiographs, whether periapical, panoramic, or CBCT, are required to interpret the entire image.

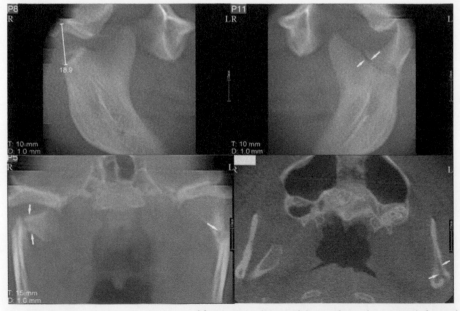

Fig. 24. The arrows point to the lines of fracture in the condylar neck on the sagittal, frontal and axial views.

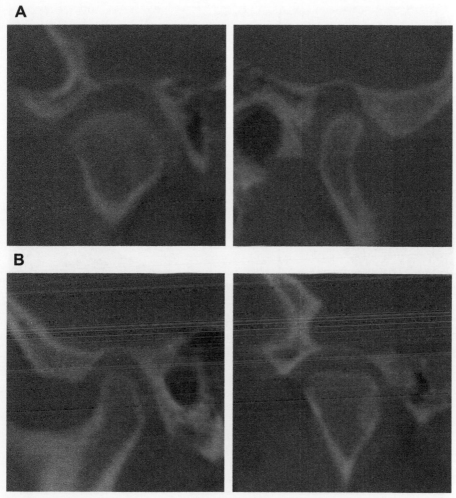

Fig. 25. (A) *Right TMJ*: Centered condyle in the glenoid fossa, in the frontal plane. Protruded downward position of the condyle in the glenoid fossa, in the sagittal plane. (B) *Left TMJ*: Centered condyle in the glenoid fossa, in the frontal plane. Centered position of the condyle in the glenoid fossa, in the sagittal plane.

If a clinician acquires a panoramic radiograph, then they are responsible for analyzing and interpreting the entire image. The same is true for CBCT. For example, if a clinician is interested in placing implants and they need a CBCT scan for bone assessment in the implant's site or fabrication of a surgical guide, the clinician is responsible for reading the entire image volume and not only evaluating the implant's site. The clinician is liable for missing lesions for a scan he or she acquires.

If a clinician does not feel comfortable reading the entire scan because of time constraints or insufficient knowledge about pathology on CBCT examinations, he or she may need to send the scan to be read by a trained oral and maxillofacial radiologist. This practice will not only provide better care for their patients but it will also offer the clinician the peace of mind and protect them from liability.

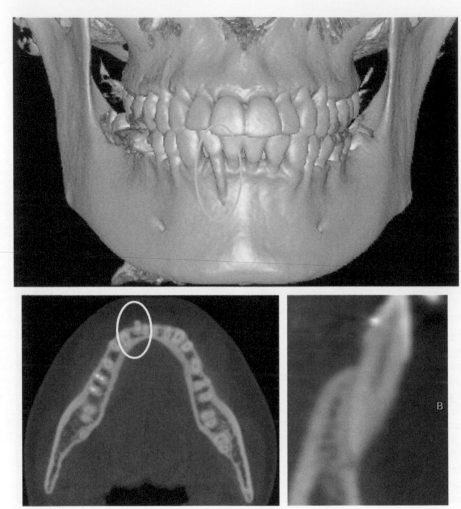

Fig. 26. Loss of the buccal plate on the lower right lateral as it appears on the 3D reconstruction (*orange circle*) and the axial view (*yellow circle*).

Clinicians who own and operate CBCT machines need to have sufficient training about best practices on how to operate their CBCT and the measures needed to acquire the best image quality scans, while at the same time lowering the radiation dose for their patients.

Clinicians are encouraged to provide adequate training for their staff; maintain proper imaging, radiation shielding, radiation records; and detect problems early on to make sure that their patients receive the best care in their practice (ALARA [As Low As Reasonably Achievable]).

Although CBCT is a useful tool in the clinician's armamentarium, it is essential that they are used when conventional means of radiography are unlikely to provide the needed information.[57]

Clinicians are encouraged to attend continuing education courses on CBCT and 3D imaging. If in need, clinicians are encouraged to ask their peers and oral and maxillofacial radiologists for help and seek their advice.

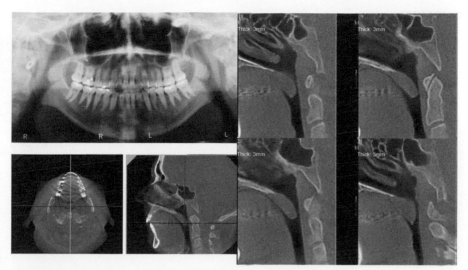

Fig. 27. Soft tissue airways as they appear on panoramic, axial, and sagittal cuts. The patient has a large soft palate.

Three-dimensional printing

In recent years, 3D printing has gained momentum because of advancements in manufacturing and materials science. From printing metal parts for automotive and aerospace to small plastic items, 3D printers are gaining market share. Cost is coming down, resolution and finishing are improving, and new materials are being developed to address different customers' needs. In addition, because the final product is not welded from different parts, this increases the product's physical properties.

In dentistry, 3D printing metal is used by dental laboratories for fabrication of metal framework for partial dentures, whereas resin printing has gained momentum for fabrication of surgical guides used for implants placements, clear aligners, and resin dentures.

Multiple manufacturers are developing 3D printers for dentistry, and dental resin can be used in some printers based on a STereoLithographic (STL) file format.

STL is a file format native to the stereolithography computer-aided design software created by 3D Systems for their first commercial printer back in the late 1980s.[58]

Dental practitioners can have the 3D printer added to their workflow in the dental office to streamline fabrication of dentures and surgical guides. Using data driven from a CBCT scan, a practitioner can plan their implant case in the software, then send the final treatment plan directly to the 3D printer using the STL format to generate a 3D printer model, a surgical guide.

Risks

As with all imaging modalities that use ionizing radiation, the use of CBCT does involve a consideration of risk to patients. However, it has the benefit of providing useful information needed to assist in making a diagnosis and/or in facilitating treatment. When a doctor refers for an x-ray examination, he or she has made the determination that the benefit outweighs the risk. One should bear in mind that the risk of most dental x-ray examinations is much less than other risks we commonly accept in daily life.

REFERENCES

1. Hounsfield GN. Computerized transverse axial scanning (tomography). 1. Description of system. Br J Radiol 1973;46:1016–22.
2. Arai Y, Tammisalo E, Iwai K, et al. Development of ortho cubic super high resolution CT (Ortho-CT). In: Lemke HU, editor. Proceedings of the 12th International Symposium and Exhibition. Tokyo, June 24–27, 1998.
3. Arai Y, Tammisalo E, Iwai K, et al. Development of a compact computed tomographic apparatus for dental use. Dentomaxillofac Radiol 1999;28(4):245–8.
4. Terakado M, Hashimoto K, Arai Y, et al. Diagnostic imaging with newly developed ortho cubic super high resolution CT (Ortho-CT). Oral Surg Oral Med Oral Pathol Oral Radiol Endod 2000;89:509–18.
5. Arai Y, Hashimoto K, Iwai K, et al. Fundamental efficiency of limited cone-beam X-ray CT (3DX multi image micro CT) for practical use. Dental Radiology 2000; 40(2):145–54.
6. Mozzo P, Procacci C, Tacconi A, et al. A new volumetric CT machine for dental imaging based on the cone-beam technique: preliminary results. Eur Radiol 1998;8(9):1558–64.
7. Scarfe WC, Farman AG. What is cone-beam CT and how does it work? Dent Clin North Am 2008;52(4):707–30.
8. Abramovitch K, Rice DD. Basic principles of cone beam computed tomography. Dent Clin North Am 2014;58(3):463–84.
9. Pauwels R, Araki K, Siewerdsen JH, et al. Technical aspects of dental CBCT: state of the art. Dentomaxillofac Radiol 2015;44(1):20140224.
10. Baba R, Konno Y, Ueda K, et al. Comparison of flat-panel detector and image-intensifier detector for cone-beam CT. Comput Med Imaging Graph 2002;26: 153–8.
11. Vano E, Geiger B, Schreiner A, et al. Dynamic flat panel detector versus image intensifier in cardiac imaging: dose and image quality. Phys Med Biol 2005;50: 5731–42.
12. Zhao Z, Gang GJ, Siewerdsen JH. Noise, sampling, and the number of projections in cone-beam CT with a flat-panel detector. Med Phys 2014;41(6):061909.
13. Kopp S, Ottl P. Dimensional stability in composite cone beam computed tomography. Dentomaxillofac Radiol 2010;39:512–6.
14. Demirturk Kocasarac H, Helvacioglu Yigit D, Bechara B, et al. Contrast-to-noise ratio with different settings in a CBCT machine in presence of different root-end filling materials: an in vitro study. Dentomaxillofac Radiol 2016;45(5):20160012.
15. Schulze RKW, Berndt D, d'Hoedt B. On cone-beam computed tomography artifacts induced by titanium implants. Clin Oral Implants Res 2010;21:100–7.
16. Pauwels R, Stamatakis H, Bosmans H, et al, The SEDENTEXCT Project Consortium. Quantification of metal artifacts on cone beam computed tomography images. Clin Oral Implants Res 2013;24(Suppl. A100):94–9.
17. Bechara B, Alex McMahan C, Moore WS, et al. Cone beam CT scans with and without artefact reduction in root fracture detection of endodontically treated teeth. Dentomaxillofac Radiol 2013;42(5):20120245.
18. Spin-Neto R, Gotfredsen E, Wenzel A. Impact of voxel size variation on CBCT-based diagnostic outcome in dentistry: a systematic review. J Digit Imaging 2013;26(4):813–20.
19. Chindasombatjaroen J, Kakimoto N, Murakami S, et al. Quantitative analysis of metallic artifacts caused by dental metals: comparison of cone-beam and multi-detector row CT scanners. Oral Radiol 2011;27(2):114–20.

20. Wang Q, Li L, Zhang L, et al. A novel metal artifact reducing method for cone-beam CT based on three approximately orthogonal projections. Phys Med Biol 2013;58(1):1–17.

21. Parsa A, Ibrahim N, Hassan B, et al. Assessment of metal artefact reduction around dental titanium implants in cone beam CT. Dentomaxillofac Radiol 2014;43(7):20140019.

22. Adibi S, Zhang W, Servos T, et al. Cone beam computed tomography in dentistry: what dental educators and learners should know. J Dent Educ 2012;76(11): 1437–42.

23. Brånemark PI. Osseointegration and its experimental background. J Prosthet Dent 1983;50(3):399–410.

24. Abraham CM. A brief historical perspective on dental implants, their surface coatings and treatments. Open Dent J 2014;8:50–5.

25. Tyndall DA, Brooks SL. Selection criteria for dental implant site imaging: a position paper of the American Academy of Oral and Maxillofacial radiology. Oral Surg Oral Med Oral Pathol Oral Radiol Endod 2000;89(5):630–7.

26. Tyndall DA, Price JB, Tetradis S, et al, American Academy of Oral and Maxillofacial Radiology. Position statement of the American Academy of Oral and Maxillofacial Radiology on selection criteria for the use of radiology in dental implantology with emphasis on cone beam computed tomography. Oral Surg Oral Med Oral Pathol Oral Radiol 2012;113(6):817–26.

27. Mah JK, Huang JC, Choo H. Practical applications of cone-beam computed tomography in orthodontics. J Am Dent Assoc 2010;141(Suppl 3).7S–13S.

28. Miracle AC, Mukherji SK. Conebeam CT of the head and neck, part 2: clinical applications. AJNR Am J Neuroradiol 2009;30(7):1285–92.

29. Kim YJ, Hong JS, Hwang YI, et al. Three-dimensional analysis of pharyngeal airway in preadolescent children with different anteroposterior skeletal patterns. Am J Orthod Dentofacial Orthop 2010;137(3):306.e1-11 [discussion: 306–7].

30. Nurko C. Three-dimensional imaging cone bean computer tomography technology: an update and case report of an impacted incisor in a mixed dentition patient. Pediatr Dent 2010;32(4):356–60.

31. Chenin DL. 3D cephalometrics: the new norm. Alpha Omegan 2010;103(2):51–6.

32. Evangelista K, Vasconcelos Kde F, Bumann A, et al. Dehiscence and fenestration in patients with class I and class II division 1 malocclusion assessed with cone-beam computed tomography. Am J Orthod Dentofacial Orthop 2010;138(2): 133.e1-7 [discussion: 133–5].

33. Wu TY, Lin HH, Lo LJ, et al. Postoperative outcomes of two- and three-dimensional planning in orthognathic surgery: a comparative study. J Plast Reconstr Aesthet Surg 2017;70(8):1101–11.

34. Kumar V, Ludlow J, Soares Cevidanes LH, et al. In vivo comparison of conventional and cone beam CT synthesized cephalograms. Angle Orthod 2008;78(5): 873–9.

35. American Academy of Oral and Maxillofacial Radiology. Clinical recommendations regarding use of cone beam computed tomography in orthodontics. [corrected]. Position statement by the American Academy of Oral and Maxillofacial Radiology. Oral Surg Oral Med Oral Pathol Oral Radiol 2013;116(2):238–57.

36. Brito-Júnior M, Quintino AF, Camilo CC, et al. Nonsurgical endodontic management using MTA for perforative defect of internal root resorption: report of a long term follow-up. Oral Surg Oral Med Oral Pathol Oral Radiol Endod 2010; 110(6):784–8.

37. Scarfe WC, Levin MD, Gane D, et al. Use of cone beam computed tomography in endodontics. Int J Dent 2009;2009:634567.
38. American Association of Endodontists, American Academy of Oral and Maxillofacial Radiology. Use of cone-beam computed tomography in endodontics joint position statement of the American Association of Endodontists and the American Academy of Oral and Maxillofacial Radiology. Oral Surg Oral Med Oral Pathol Oral Radiol Endod 2011;111(2):234–7.
39. Fayad MI, Nair M, Levin MD, et al. Special committee to revise the joint AAE/AAOMR position statement on use of CBCT in endodontics. AAE and AAOMR joint position statement: use of cone beam computed tomography in endodontics 2015 update. Oral Surg Oral Med Oral Pathol Oral Radiol 2015;120(4):508–12.
40. Jaju PP, Jaju SP. Clinical utility of dental cone-beam computed tomography: current perspectives. Clin Cosmet Investig Dent 2014;6:29–43.
41. Bortoluzzi MC, Manfro R. Treatment for ectopic third molar in the subcondylar region planned with cone beam computed tomography: a case report. J Oral Maxillofac Surg 2010;68(4):870–2.
42. Rege IC, Sousa TO, Leles CR, et al. Occurrence of maxillary sinus abnormalities detected by cone beam CT in asymptomatic patients. BMC Oral Health 2012;12:30.
43. Zhou HH, Ongodia D, Liu Q, et al. Dental trauma in patients with maxillofacial fractures. Dent Traumatol 2013;29(4):285–90.
44. Pickrell BB, Hollier LH Jr. Evidence-based medicine: mandible fractures. Plast Reconstr Surg 2017;140(1):192e–200e.
45. Kaeppler G, Cornelius CP, Ehrenfeld M, et al. Diagnostic efficacy of cone-beam computed tomography for mandibular fractures. Oral Surg Oral Med Oral Pathol Oral Radiol 2013;116(1):98–104.
46. Bae S, Park MS, Han JW, et al. Correlation between pain and degenerative bony changes on cone-beam computed tomography images of temporomandibular joints. Maxillofac Plast Reconstr Surg 2017;39(1):19.
47. Caruso S, Storti E, Nota A, et al. Temporomandibular joint anatomy assessed by CBCT images. Biomed Res Int 2017;2017:2916953.
48. Summa S, Ursini R, Manicone PF, et al. MRI assessment of temporomandibular disorders: an approach to diagnostic and therapeutic setting. Cranio 2014;32(2):131–8.
49. Al-Saleh MA, Alsufyani NA, Saltaji H, et al. MRI and CBCT image registration of temporomandibular joint: a systematic review. J Otolaryngol Head Neck Surg 2016;45(1):30.
50. Guo YJ, Ge ZP, Ma RH, et al. A six-site method for the evaluation of periodontal bone loss in cone-beam CT images. Dentomaxillofac Radiol 2016;45(1):20150265.
51. de Faria Vasconcelos K, Evangelista KM, Rodrigues CD, et al. Detection of periodontal bone loss using cone beam CT and intraoral radiography. Dentomaxillofac Radiol 2012;41:64–9.
52. Goodarzi Pour D, Romoozi E, Soleimani Shayesteh Y. Accuracy of cone beam computed tomography for detection of bone loss. J Dent (Tehran) 2015;12(7):513–23.
53. Ramesh R, Sadasivan A. Oral squamous cell carcinoma masquerading as gingival overgrowth. Eur J Dent 2017;11(3):390–4.
54. Zinsly SDR, Moraes LC, Moura P, et al. Assessment of pharyngeal airway space using cone-beam computed tomography. Dental Press J Orthod 2010;15(5):150–8.

55. Grauer D, Cevidanes LS, Styner MA, et al. Pharyngeal airway volume and shape from cone-beam computed tomography: relationship to facial morphology. Am J Orthod Dentofacial Orthop 2009;136(6):805–14.
56. American Dental Association Council on Scientific Affairs. The use of cone-beam computed tomography in dentistry: an advisory statement from the American Dental Association Council on Scientific Affairs. J Am Dent Assoc 2012;143(8): 899–902.
57. Merrett SJ, Drage NA, Durning P. Cone beam computed tomography: a useful tool in orthodontic diagnosis and treatment planning. J Orthod 2009;36(3): 202–10.
58. Chakravorty D. STL file format for 3D printing - simply explained. All3DP. 2017. Available at: https://all3dp.com. Accessed March 30, 2018.

3D Volume Rendering and 3D Printing (Additive Manufacturing)

Rujuta A. Katkar, BDS, MDS, MS[a],*, Robert M. Taft, DDS[b],
Gerald T. Grant, DMD, MS[c]

KEYWORDS

- 3D printing • 3D volume rendering • Additive manufacturing • Rapid prototyping

KEY POINTS

- Three-dimensional (3D) volume rendering can be useful in volumetric assessment of bone defects; however, this still needs to be visualized on a computer monitor.
- 3D printing, additive manufacturing, and rapid prototyping techniques are being used in surgical planning with satisfactory accuracy.
- Categories of additive manufacturing techniques are discussed based on manufacturing process.
- 3D printing applications in dentistry and maxillofacial prosthetics are discussed.
- Limitations include time and cost; accuracy depends on type of 3D printer, material, and build thickness.

THREE-DIMENSIONAL VOLUME RENDERING

Volume rendering is a set of techniques used to display a 2-dimensional (D) projection of a 3D discretely sampled data set. These volume-rendered images can be sectioned in any plane and rotated in space, allowing 3D insight into the anatomy of craniofacial bones. 3D-rendered images provide additional information for surgical planning and teaching. Both multislice computed tomography and cone beam computed tomography (CBCT) have been shown as reliable techniques in the volumetric assessment of bone defects in alveolar and palatal regions.[1] With these techniques, accurate assessment of the size and extent of bone defects caused by oral clefts, for example, is possible. This is important not only in the treatment planning but also to establish

Disclosure Statement: The authors have nothing to disclose.
[a] Department of Comprehensive Dentistry, University of Texas Health San Antonio, School of Dentistry, 7703 Floyd Curl Drive, San Antonio, TX 78229-3900, USA; [b] Department of Comprehensive Dentistry, University of Texas Health San Antonio, School of Dentistry, MC 7914, 7703 Floyd Curl Drive, San Antonio, TX 78229-3900, USA; [c] Oral Health and Rehabilitation, University of Louisville School of Dentistry, 501 South Preston Street, Room 311, Louisville, KY 40202, USA
* Corresponding author.
E-mail address: katkarr@uthscsa.edu

Dent Clin N Am 62 (2018) 393–402
https://doi.org/10.1016/j.cden.2018.03.003
0011-8532/18/© 2018 Elsevier Inc. All rights reserved.

the donor area and the volume of bone graft (**Fig. 1**). However, these volume-rendered images are still limited to viewing on a computer monitor and provide only additional visual cues. For a novice surgeon with limited experience with spatial perception, accurately evaluating the anatomy from visual cues alone may be cognitively and perceptually demanding. Consequently, 3D-rendered images may not provide a significant advantage over traditional visualization methods.[2]

3D PRINTING OR ADDITIVE MANUFACTURING

3D printing, also known as additive manufacturing and rapid prototyping, was first developed in late 1980s and was soon applied in medicine and surgery. The application of digital technology with 3D volumetric imaging was first introduced to the craniomaxillofacial region in 1983.[3] In the 1990s, computer-aided design and computer-aided manufacturing techniques began to be used in craniomaxillofacial surgery. Many reports have demonstrated satisfactory accuracy of 3D-printed models generated from DICOM® (Digital Imaging and Communications in Medicine) images and their use in surgical treatment planning.[4–10]

Additive manufacturing technologies have been categorized by the American Society for Testing and Materials Standards body (ASTM Active Standard F2792, June 2012) according to manufacturing process (**Fig. 2**):

- Vat polymerization: Based on the exposure of a light source to a vat of a light-sensitive resin in a layered fashion. Examples used in dentistry are stereolithography or directed light projection. This type of printing requires a fair amount of post processing to remove supports, remove unused material, and to complete the cure of the material. These types of printers have become popular in dentistry (**Figs. 3–5**).
- Materials extrusion: Use of a filament that is extruded through a heated extruder of a known diameter. This is the technology in most of the inexpensive desktop printers used by hobbyists; however, it does have some application in dental and medical use for models. This also has some necessary postprocessing.
- Material jetting: Use of a material that is jetted through multiple ports, the material is then cured layer by layer. This permits use of different materials that allow for color or different durometer (stiffness) within the same print. Supports are generally easily removed and the print is completed
- Binder jetting: A bed of powder, generally a gypsum material. A print head delivers color and a binder layer by layer. The powder supports the piece. The completed part generally needs some type of postprocessing because the part is rather fragile.

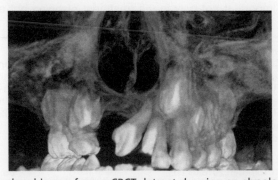

Fig. 1. Volume-rendered image from a CBCT dataset showing an alveolar cleft defect.

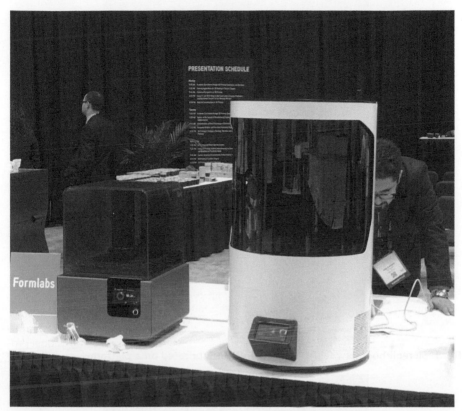

Fig. 2. Commercially available directed light projection printers are classified as vat polymerization types. These current laptop printers (NewPro 3D, Vancouver, Canada; Formlabs, Somerville, MA) provide the flexibility of materials available.

- Powder bed fusion: Different powders, from metals, nylons, and other polymers are fused with a laser or electron beam source. This technology requires a fair amount of postprocessing and is used for printing cobalt chrome and titanium frameworks for fixed and removable prosthetics in dentistry.
- Direct energy deposition: A powder flows directly under a source, such as a laser, and the material is placed as needed. This is very useful in repair of a metal part.
- Sheet lamination: A sheet of material is stacked with a binder as the outline is cut away with each layer. The resolution depends on the thickness of the sheet.

The fabrication of 3D-printed models (biomodels) for diagnosis, surgical training, and planning seem to be the most common uses of additive technology, followed by application for direct manufacture of implantable devices.[11] In maxillofacial surgery, printing a model based on scans of the area of interest allows for more thorough preplanning of complex cases and the ability to test fit the fabricated parts before the procedure (**Fig. 6**). This has been to shown to lead to an increase in fit accuracy of fabricated prostheses and a reduction in operative time by 30 to 90 minutes.[12] Furthermore, customized cranial reconstruction implant prostheses are required when treating large cranial defects. The use of custom titanium implants, fabricated using direct metal laser sintering additive technology, for such defects has been demonstrated to be much quicker to fabricate and place during surgery than conventional methods.

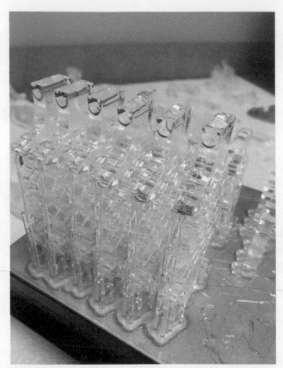

Fig. 3. Stereolithography fabricated test coupons fabricated on a platform.

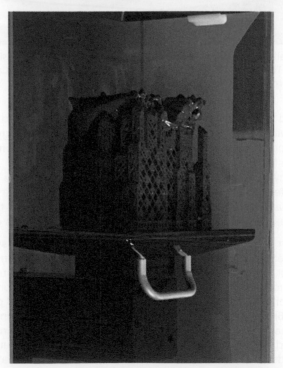

Fig. 4. Because 3D printers provide an active layer, usually with minimally cured material, structures are used to support model parts that generally exceed 30° from upright positions.

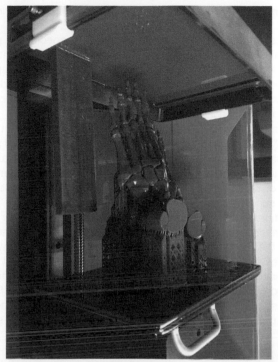

Fig. 5. Newer print strategies allow for stereolithography and directed light projection sources to use small vats and build within the vat and excess resin removed with each layer.

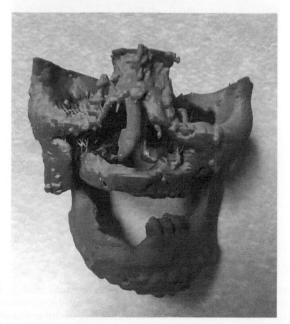

Fig. 6. A complex anatomic model.

This is due to high accuracy and the ease in which various modifications are made to suit each case at the design stage.[13]

Advances in preoperative virtual planning and patient-specific 3D printing seem to provide additional predictability in complex surgical cases. A recent study reported that the quality of preoperative planning for novice surgeons is improved with the use of 3D-printed models when compared with 3D volume-rendered images in pancreatic surgery.[2] However, no such comparative study was found for the dental and maxillofacial region in a literature search.

The major limitation of rapid prototyping lies in time and cost spent in generation of 3D objects (**Fig. 7**). Widespread use of rapid prototyping for surgical planning or individual implant design does not seem to be justified because standard planning procedures or standard implants are sufficient. However, in complicated cases, additional costs of rapid prototyping may be compensated by reduced operating times and higher success rate of the surgical procedure.[14]

3D printing techniques are often presented as a timesaving tool for use in the operating room; however, this alleged advantage is often counterbalanced by the time spent to prepare the model. According to a recent systematic review on advantages and disadvantages of 3D printing in surgery, most of the reported studies were in hospital-based maxillofacial (50.0%) and orthopedic (24.7%) operations. The main advantages reported were the possibilities for preoperative planning (48.7%), the accuracy of the process used (33.5%), and the time saved in the operating room (32.9%); however, 21.5% of the studies stressed that the accuracy was not satisfactory. The

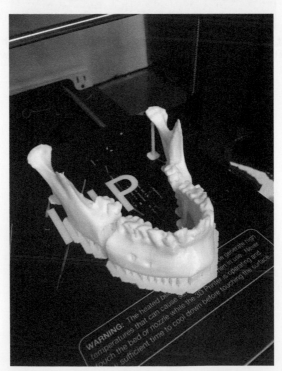

Fig. 7. Filament deposition modeling can be useful for medical models. It is inexpensive: many of the printers can be purchased for less than $1000 and the filament is inexpensive. However, the process is very slow and, owing to the nature of the preparation of the build, it is best used when only the surface is of importance.

time needed to prepare the object (19.6%) and the additional costs (19.0%) were also seen as important limitations for routine use of 3D printing. Most of these studies were case reports and case series with only 1 randomized controlled trial. The number of advantages reported on 3D printing was twice that of reported disadvantages; however, this could be due to a publication bias with some investigators or journal editors being reluctant to publish negative findings.[15]

To establish evidence-based guidelines, it will be essential to know in which types of maxillofacial surgery and reconstruction. 3D printing is better than standard imaging with or without volume rendering. This might have an impact on the reimbursement for 3D-printed models.

Also, a 3D-printed skull model of the same individual can vary markedly depending on the DICOM® to STL (stereolithography) conversion software and the technical parameters used. In a recent study, a large variation was noted in size and anatomic geometries of the 3 physical skull models fabricated from an identical (or a single) DICOM® data set derived from a CBCT scan. Clinicians should be aware of this inaccuracy in certain applications.[16] Threshold-based segmentations can vary extensively and are, therefore, likely to be a potential source of error in biomodeling. Even though the approximate radiodensity ranges of typical tissues are known, a certain amount of subjective consideration is required when choosing the threshold intensity value. This problem is especially evident when the voxel intensity distribution over the image is nonuniform, such as in CBCT imaging, and the image is not properly corrected.[16]

Three-Dimensional Printing in Dentistry

The basic premise of digital workflow in dentistry is based around 3 elements. First is data acquisition, such as in various scanning technologies. This is followed by manipulation and processing of data, created using a computer-aided design software. Finally, the processed data are used for manufacturing of structures in the desired material through computer-aided manufacturing.[17] In the manufacturing step, 3D printing (additive manufacturing) is becoming a fast growing alternative for certain manufacturing previously performed by subtractive manufacturing.

3D printing technology is being used in various dental applications, primarily in implant dentistry for making surgical guides. In implantology, the use of surgical guides has been strongly recommended to facilitate better planning and reduce the risk of operative complications.[18] The accuracy of surgical guides produced using stereolithography has been shown to be fairly accurate, with an angular deviation of 2° and linear deviation of 1.1 mm at the hex and 2 mm at the apex.[19] The fabrication of custom implant screws has also been researched. The SLS additive process can create implants with complex geometry and a porous surface. This has been shown to increase osseointegration and has been successfully tested in patients.[20,21]

The type of 3D printer, material used for printing, and build thickness are known to influence the accuracy of printed models. Fleming and colleagues[22] reviewed studies that compared conventional and digital dental models. They found varying reported results but minimal differences, and seemed to advocate the differences as clinically acceptable. However, data distortion during data conversion and manipulation to convert the digital surface information to the stereolithography file format, and the subsequent model shrinkage during building and postcuring from the rapid prototyping technique, may further influence the accuracy of the reconstructed models.[23] One recent study compared reconstructed rapid prototyping models produced by 3D printing and conventional stone models for different degrees of dental crowding. Statistically significant differences were found for all planes in all categories of crowding, except for crown height in the moderate crowding group and arch dimensions in the

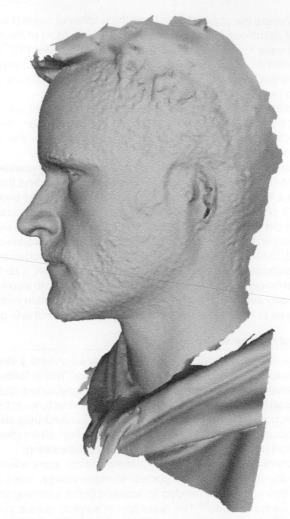

Fig. 8. Capture of patient defect from a digital camera system. An STL file can be fabricated for design and fabrication of the ear either from the contralateral side or from a library.

mild and moderate crowding groups. It was concluded that the rapid prototyping models were not clinically comparable with conventional stone models regardless of the degree of crowding.[23]

Additive manufacturing is being used and investigated for several intraoral prosthodontic applications, including printing stone models from intraoral scans, making custom impression trays, and direct fabrication of dental prostheses.[24,25]

The use of additive manufacturing is also being investigated in bone graft applications with customizable scaffold material, allowing for control of overall hardness and rate of dissolution.[26]

In maxillofacial prosthetics, the combination of scanning technology, design software, and 3D printers allow for a much more comfortable digital impression technique and prosthesis fabrication. Extraoral prosthesis fabrication has proven to be useful in pediatric restorations. With minimal capture times, use of digital design, and printing molds a prosthesis can be fabricated with very little interaction with the patient.[27]

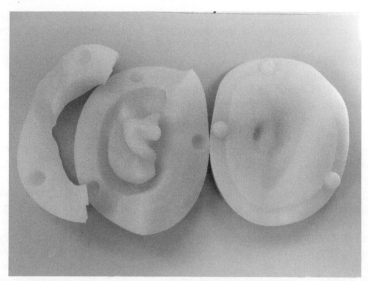

Fig. 9. 3D-printed mold for an ear.

These technologies provide access to fabrication of extraoral prosthesis in cases in which there is minimum support to provide the expertise for the traditional sculpting and mold fabrication. Digital images can be downloaded to a commercial vender and design can be done remotely through virtual meetings (**Figs. 8** and **9**).

REFERENCES

1. Albuquerque MA, Gaia BF, Cavalcanti MGP. Comparison between multislice and cone-beam computerized tomography in the volumetric assessment of cleft palate. Oral Surg Oral Med Oral Pathol Oral Radiol Endod 2011;112:249–57.
2. Zheng Y, Yu D, Zhao J, et al. 3D printout models vs. 3D-rendered images: which is better for preoperative planning? J Surg Educ 2016;73:518–23.
3. Hemmy D, David D, Herman G. Three-dimensional reconstruction of craniofacial deformity using computed tomography. Neurosurgery 1983;13:534–41.
4. D'Urso PS, Barker TM, Earwaker WJ, et al. Stereolithographic biomodelling in cranio-maxillofacial surgery: a prospective trial. J Craniomaxillofac Surg 1999; 27:30–7.
5. Zhou L, Shang H, He L, et al. Accurate reconstruction of discontinuous mandible using a reverse Engineering/Computer-aided Design/Rapid prototyping technique: a preliminary clinical study. J Oral Maxillofac Surg 2010;68:2115–21.
6. Zimmerer RM, Ellis E III, Aniceto GS, et al. A prospective multicenter study to compare the precision of posttraumatic internal orbital reconstruction with standard preformed and individualized orbital implants. J Craniomaxillofac Surg 2016;44:1485–97.
7. Arora A, Datarkar AN, Borle RM, et al. Custom-made implant for maxillofacial defects using rapid prototype models. J Oral Maxillofac Surg 2013;71:e104–10.
8. Taft RM, Kondor S, Grant GT. Accuracy of rapid prototype models for head and neck reconstruction. J Prosthet Dent 2011;106:399–408.
9. Nizam A, Gopal R, Naing L, et al. Dimensional accuracy of the skull models produced by rapid prototyping technology using stereolithography apparatus. Arch Orofac Sci 2006;1:60–1, 66.

10. Salmi M, Paloheimo KS, Tuomi J, et al. Accuracy of medical models made by additive manufacturing (rapid manufacturing). J Craniomaxillofac Surg 2013;41: 603–9.
11. Lantada AD, Morgado PL. Rapid prototyping for biomedical engineering: current capabilities and challenges. Annu Rev Biomed Eng 2012;14:73–96.
12. Wilde F, Plail M, Riese C, et al. Mandible reconstruction with patient-specific prebent reconstruction plates: comparison of a transfer key method to the standard method–results of an in vitro study. Int J Comput Assist Radiol Surg 2012;7: 57–63.
13. Jardini AL, Larosa MA, Filho RM, et al. Cranial reconstruction: 3D biomodel and custom-built implant created using additive manufacturing. J Craniomaxillofac Surg 2014;42:1877–84.
14. Rengier F, Mehndiratta A, von Tengg-Kobligk H, et al. 3D printing based on imaging data: Review of medical applications. Int J Comput Assist Radiol Surg 2010;5: 335–41.
15. Martelli N, Serrano C, van den Brink H, et al. Advantages and disadvantages of 3-dimensional printing in surgery: a systematic review. Surgery 2016;159:1485–500.
16. Huotilainen E, Jaanimets R, Valášek J, et al. Inaccuracies in additive manufactured medical skull models caused by the DICOM to STL conversion process. J Craniomaxillofac Surg 2014;42:e259–65.
17. van Noort R. The future of dental devices is digital. Dental Mater 2012;28:3–12.
18. Lal K, White GS, Morea DN, et al. Use of stereolithographic templates for surgical and prosthodontic implant planning and placement. Part I. the concept. J Prosthodont 2006;15:51–8.
19. Turbush SK, Turkyilmaz I. Accuracy of three different types of stereolithographic surgical guide in implant placement: an in vitro study. J Prosthet Dent 2012;108: 181–8.
20. Figliuzzi M, Mangano F, Mangano C. A novel root analogue dental implant using CT scan and CAD/CAM: selective laser melting technology. Int J Oral Maxillofac Surg 2012;41:858–62.
21. Mangano FG, De Franco M, Caprioglio A, et al. Immediate, non-submerged, root-analogue direct laser metal sintering (DLMS) implants: a 1-year prospective study on 15 patients. Lasers Med Sci 2014;29:1321–8.
22. Fleming P, Marinho V, Johal A. Orthodontic measurements on digital study models compared with plaster models: a systematic review. Orthod Craniofac Res 2011;14:1–16.
23. Wan Hassan WN, Yusoff Y, Mardi NA. Comparison of reconstructed rapid prototyping models produced by 3-dimensional printing and conventional stone models with different degrees of crowding. Am J Orthod Dentofacial Orthop 2017;151:209–18.
24. Barazanchi A, Li KC, Al-Amleh B, et al. Additive technology: update on current materials and applications in dentistry. J Prosthodont 2017;26(2):156–63.
25. Chen H, Zhao T, Wang Y, et al. Computer aided design and 3-dimensional printing for the production of custom trays of maxillary edentulous jaws based on 3-dimensional scan of primary impression. Beijing Da Xue Xue Bao Yi Xue Ban 2016;48:900–4.
26. Habibovic P, Gbureck U, Doillon CJ, et al. Osteoconduction and osteoinduction of low-temperature 3D printed bioceramic implants. Biomaterials 2008;29:944–53.
27. Grant GT, Aita-Holmes C, Liacouras P, et al. Digital capture, design and manufacturing of an facial prosthesis: clinical report on pediatric patient. J Prosthet Dent 2015;114(1):138–41.

Computer-Assisted Surgery
Applications in Dentistry and Oral and Maxillofacial Surgery

Carlos G. Landaeta-Quinones, DDS*, Nicole Hernandez, DDS, MD,
Najy K. Zarroug, DDS, MD

KEYWORDS

- Computer-assisted navigation • Virtual surgical planning • Intraoperative navigation

KEY POINTS

- Computer-assisted surgery (CAS) has great utility in implant dentistry as well as cranio-maxillofacial surgery.
- Computer-assisted surgery (CAS) allows the surgeon to precisely plan and execute complex surgical treatment in an efficient manner.
- The future and direction of CAS will allow the surgeon in the near future to complete more complex procedures, improving accuracy, and ultimately reducing patient time in the chair.

INTRODUCTION

Computer-assisted surgery (CAS) has evolved over time from its origins in the late 1800s as stereotaxy, which was used to obtain cerebral biopsies in neurosurgical procedures. A few years later, in the first decade of the twentieth century, Horsley and Clarke devised a method for using a head frame in combination with a stereotactic atlas. CAS has evolved from framed to frameless stereotaxy, to currently using optical tracking. The first navigation system based on an optical instrument presented in the early 1990s by Heilbrunn and colleagues.[1] Currently, computer navigation uses optical tracking, which can be categorized as active or passive optical systems. It has gained popularity in dentistry and craniomaxillofacial (CMF) surgery within the last 20 years. There is currently a positive role for CAS in implantology and oral and maxillofacial surgery (OMS), including orthognathic and temporomandibular joint (TMJ) surgery, facial trauma, maxillomandibular reconstruction.

Disclosure Statement: The authors have nothing to disclose.
UT Dentistry-Oral and Maxillofacial Surgery, 8210 Floyd Curl Drive, San Antonio, TX 78229, USA
* Corresponding author.
E-mail address: landaeta@uthscsa.edu

Dent Clin N Am 62 (2018) 403–420
https://doi.org/10.1016/j.cden.2018.03.009
0011-8532/18/© 2018 Elsevier Inc. All rights reserved.

dental.theclinics.com

The ability to visualize the patient in 3 dimensions is an important aspect of successful dental surgery. CAS allows the clinician to visualize the patient in the sagittal, coronal, and axial planes on a computer workstation, and to construct several virtual plans in conjunction with a design engineer. By using computerized technology, the clinician today has the capability of obtaining increasing accuracy in placement of dental implants, bone grafts, and hardware, as well as tumor excision, while concurrently reducing the risk of iatrogenic injury or suboptimal surgical outcomes.

Computer-aided design and computer-aided manufacturing (CAD/CAM) have historically been used in dentistry as a tool for dental implants and restorative prostheses. Digital impressions and restorations can be fabricated and delivered in a single visit. This eliminates the need for multiple visits and improves accuracy by reducing conventional errors. Digital impressions are particularly useful in patients with hyperactive gag reflexes and limited mouth opening that make conventional diagnostic impressions difficult to obtain.

CAS is currently used for virtual surgical planning (VSP), intraoperative navigation (static and dynamic), and intraoperative postsurgical computer tomography (CT) and/or MRI.[2] The intent of this article is to discuss the indications of CAS in dentistry and its subspecialties such as OMS, implantology, and prosthodontics. It highlights the process, benefits, and shortcomings of each modality; presents cases pertaining to each area of application; and explores the future of CAS.

PROCESS

The process of CAS begins with data acquisition (**Fig. 1**). A preoperative CT scan of the patient is obtained, which is then converted into a digital imaging and communications in medicine (DICOM) format. The DICOM data can be used in several ways, including creating 3-dimensional (3D) stereolithic (STL) models, performing virtual surgical simulations (with VSP), and navigating intraoperatively.

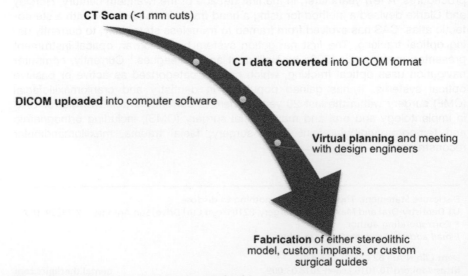

CT Scan (<1 mm cuts)

CT data converted into DICOM format

DICOM uploaded into computer software

Virtual planning and meeting with design engineers

Fabrication of either stereolithic model, custom implants, or custom surgical guides

Fig. 1. The general process and order involved in CAS.

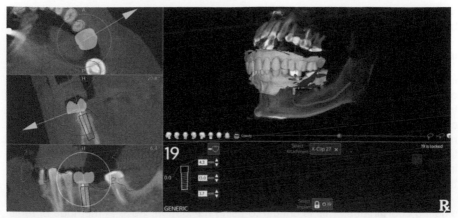

Fig. 2. Implant planning software illustrating VSP of implant at site #20. The position of the inferior alveolar nerve is clearly outlined to minimize risk of injury, the implant angulation can be manipulated and visualized in all 3 dimensions.

PRESURGICAL PLANNING

Traditional surgical planning has been associated with an extended period of time. Computer-assisted surgical planning can reduce the amount of time required while simultaneously decreasing error and improving esthetic results (**Fig. 2**).

In addition, another computer planning modality commonly used in dentistry and OMS is stereolithography, which uses CT datasets to create STL models. STL models have been used in the past as templates to prebend fixation hardware in cases of mandibular resections and reconstructions, for planning margins in tumor ablations, and to fabricate custom implants (**Fig. 3**). The technology available today offers the ability to create a digital plan for ablative surgery and specific tumor margins, as well as obviating the need for free-handed prebending for the restoration of bony defects. This minimizes possible iatrogenic injury to nearby structures such as the inferior alveolar nerve, as well as pre-determining which teeth may be compromised from resection margins. Actions such as segmentation of certain structures,

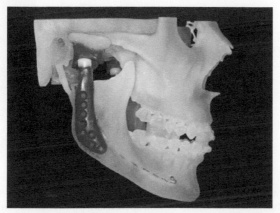

Fig. 3. Preoperative STL model created from DICOM dataset of patient for fabrication of custom TMJ prosthesis with planned condylectomies and coronoidectomies.

mirror imaging, implant positioning, and addition of structures are possible with VSP based on DICOM data.[2]

INTRAOPERATIVE NAVIGATION

Intraoperative navigation enables the clinician to see the placement of his instrument on the 3D dataset of the patient during real-time surgery. The process involves optical tracking by 2 distinct methods: (1) active and (2) passive. Active systems use infrared cameras to detect light-emitting diodes to perform instrument tracking. On the other hand, passive systems rely on reflectors rather than light sources for instrument tracking, which eliminates the need for batteries or electrical cords.[1] A tracking device is attached to the patient and detected by the camera, which then triangulates the patient's anatomic position into the virtual software (**Fig. 4**).

Registration refers to merging the CT scan coordinates to the patient's actual existing coordinates. This is critical to using navigation. Several methods of registration are available, including point registration, surface registration, and hybrid registration.[3] Point registration is the standard method due in part to the high level of accuracy and low target registration error. Both the patient's postoperative registration and the presurgical plan can later be merged in the software. Most clinicians can attest to a successful virtually guided surgical outcome if it falls within 2 mm of the planned predictions.[4] Registration of the points is critical, and improper registration can lead to inaccuracies in the final surgical outcomes. Both the patient's registration and the presurgical plan can later be merged in the software. Several studies have proved this technology to be precise, effective, and time efficient.[3]

APPLICATIONS
Dental Implants

The traditional method for placing implants has been to insert them freehand or guided by using a laboratory-made surgical stent created from diagnostic impressions. CAS

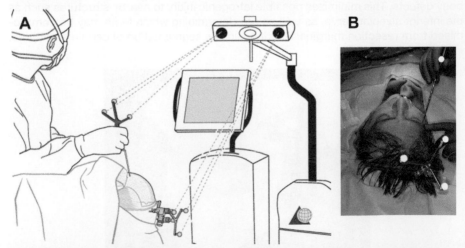

Fig. 4. (A) The point registration method using optical tracking array attached to patient's head. (B) Patient with right orbital floor fracture. Intraoperatively, point registration was performed to confirm the preplanned landmarks with the patient's intraoperative anatomy. (*From* AO Surgery Reference, www.aosurgery.org. Copyright by AO Foundation, Switzerland.)

can be used in implant dentistry for the following modalities using the patient's preoperative cone beam CT (CBCT):

1. 3D planning of implant position
2. Fabrication of static implant guides
3. Fully guided dynamic navigation.

There are manufacturers that have developed CAS hardware and software that help make dental implant insertion more accurate. Static CAS systems use drill guides fabricated with CAD/CAM based on the VSP. In addition, dynamic implant placement is possible in which the drill is optically tracked (**Fig. 5**). This offers real-time positioning and instrument guidance, which can be visualized on the digital workstation (**Fig. 6**).

There are several indications for using CT-guided static guides for implant dentistry. For example, in an esthetic area in which a flapless approach may be desired, a VSP-generated stent can be used for accurate angulation and depth. Certain cases, including full arch rehabilitation with implants and fixed prostheses can benefit by the use of VSP-guided stents to reduce intraoperative time while improving the accuracy of the implant placement (**Fig. 7**).[5] This benefits the surgeon as well as the restorative dentist.

Dynamic navigation in implant dentistry has great utility in certain case settings. For example, in cases with limited mouth opening, the use of bulky surgical guides is not possible. Therefore, by using the technology of digital presurgical planning in conjunction with navigation, the clinician can eliminate the need for a surgical guide and can

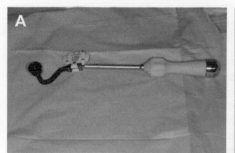
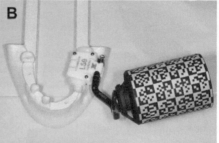
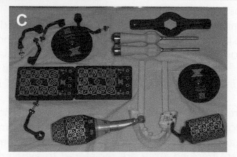

Fig. 5. X-Nav Dynamic Navigation for Implants. (*A*) Custom X-clip, which is placed onto teeth with 3 fiducial markers and with connection for patient tracker. (*B, C*) Complete armamentarium for dynamic implant navigation consisting of patient X-clip, patient tracking device, and tracking device for surgical handpiece. Also shown are the calibration plates for the system. The patient tracker attaches to the X-clip. (*Courtesy of* X-Nav Technologies, Lansdale, PA.)

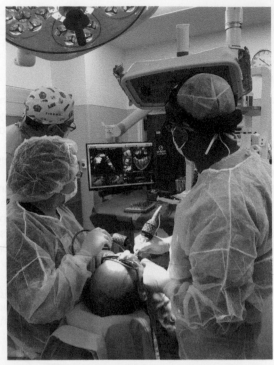

Fig. 6. Workstation with receiver and monitor illustrating the clinician's position of optically tracked implant drill in real time superimposed on the virtual plan. The clinician focuses attention on the screen to guide the direction of the handpiece based on the virtual plan.

determine its implant location based on the real-time navigation (**Fig. 8**). Similarly, dynamic navigation is helpful in cases with poor visualization of the surgical field. Using dynamic navigation versus static navigation allows the clinician to place accurate implants on the same day as the CT imaging is obtained by eliminating the need to fabricate a surgical guide. Finally, dynamic navigation helps the clinician to identify the exact location of adjacent teeth and/or vital structures. This enables optimal safety during implant placement and allows for determination of dimensions necessary for restorations and prostheses.

In regard to dynamic navigation, scanning protocols exist for dentate patients, all of which begin with the jaw registration. This consists of transferring the patient information into the navigation software using a clip with 3 metallic fiducial markers adapted to the teeth using heat.[5,6] The clips are placed on the contralateral side of the same jaw that will receive the implant to avoid the surgical field. A CBCT is then obtained with the device in place.

Virtual implants are then placed with restorative and space considerations in mind using a software program. The implant length, width, and platform are entered into the database to replicate exact geometric measurements. On the day of surgery, the handpiece and patient tracking array are registered to synchronize the real patient with the virtual patient. The surgeon then performs the surgery with each implant drill length calibrated. It is very important to continue to check the accuracy of the tracking array to avoid errors. The surgeon focuses her or his attention on the navigation screen rather than on the patient. The software shows the angulation, position, and depth of the drill in real time (**Fig. 9**).

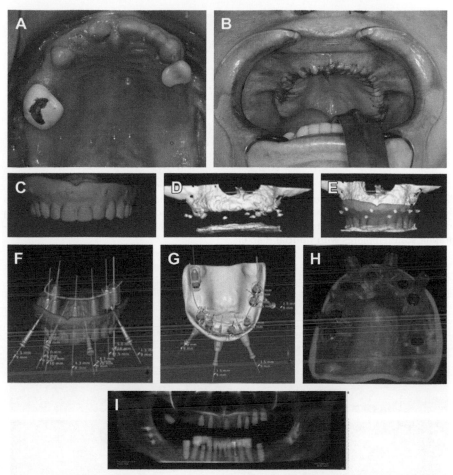

Fig. 7. A case of static navigation for dental implants with planned maxillary fixed prosthesis. (*A*) Non-restorable maxillary dentition. The patient desired an implant-retained fixed prosthesis and, therefore, underwent extractions of remaining maxillary teeth (*B*). (*C, D*) The dual-scan technique was used, beginning with CBCT of maxillary denture marked with radiopaque markers. (*E*) Merging of patient's scanned denture with fiduciary markers. The denture is then inserted in the patient and a new scan is obtained. (*F, G*) The data from the 2 scans are then merged to develop the virtual plan for implant placement. (*H*) Custom surgical guide with positioning screws used intraoperatively to guide angulation and depth of implant. (*I*) Postoperative panorex of final implant placement.

Several advantages are offered by using CAS for implant placement, whether using drill guides or dynamic navigation. This includes accurate depth control, which can result in decreased risk of damage to vital structures. CAS also provides the ability to perform flapless or limited flap elevation. Finally, it is helpful in performing accurate spacing and angulation, which results in improved esthetic outcomes.

Despite these advantages, there are a few disadvantages to the use of static navigation. In cases of static guides for implant placement, the position of the implant cannot be changed intraoperatively from the virtually created surgical guide. Also, it

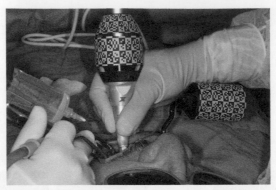

Fig. 8. The tracking process of moving objects for implant placement consists of mounting a dynamic reference frame on the patient using the following methods: bone markers using microscrews, external registration with fiducial markers, and dentures fixed with radiographic scan templates with fiducial markers.

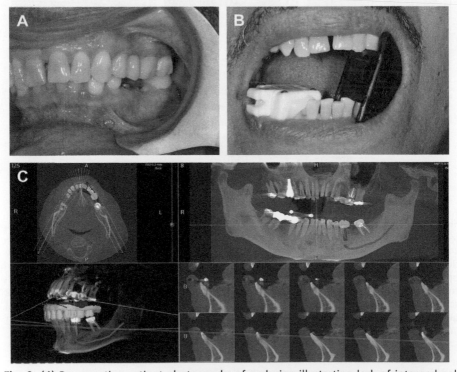

Fig. 9. (*A*) Preoperative patient photographs of occlusion illustrating lack of interocclusal space. (*B*) X-Nav clipped onto patient's teeth on right side in preparation for implant at site #20. (*C*) Implant planning software used to plan ideal dental implant and restorative crown positioning. In addition, the positioning of the inferior alveolar nerve, as well as the planned angulation in the axial and sagittal views (coronal views not shown). The virtual plan can be used intraoperatively with navigation systems to confirm the predetermined placement. Planning and fabrication of the ideal size of the crown in all 3 dimensions is facilitated with use of virtual software. (*D*) Dynamic handpiece used to place implant according to predetermined angulation. (*E*) Final implant at site #20. Images (*F-H*) demonstrating the final implant position at site #20 in 3 planes of view on CT Max/face as well as final panorex image.

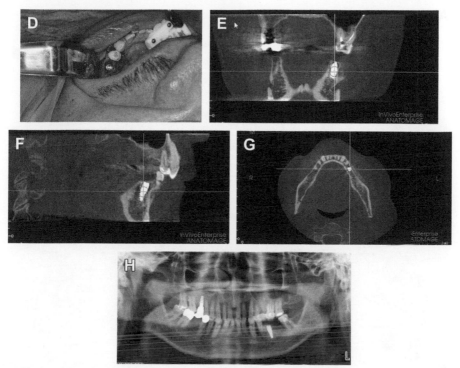

Fig. 9. (*continued*).

is challenging to irrigate the drill throughout the procedure, which increases the risk of bone necrosis and implant failure.[7]

When looking at the accuracy of implant placement with CAS, a large prospective cohort study found that freehand implant placement had significantly greater amounts of deviation from the plan when compared with using partially or fully guided implant navigation.[2] When comparing freehand versus static navigation, the use of a static, VSP-generated guide stent with a coordinated system of specified drilling can result in less than 2 mm crestal and apical deviation from the plan, and an angulation error of less than 5°.[5] The results from studies by Chiu and colleagues, Kramer and colleagues, Brief and colleagues, and Casap and colleagues suggest that dynamic navigation systems have an entry error approximating 0.4 mm and an angular deviation error approximating 4°.[5]

Despite the increased accuracy and time efficiency offered by CAS, there are some associated disadvantages for implant placement. Due to the rather novel use of CAS implant placement, there is a variable learning curve associated with developing comfort using the system. The software requires accurate calibration. The registration template can pose difficulty if loose or misfitted, such as in edentulous patients. In can be interpreted from the study by Ganss and colleagues[5] that CAS was superior in accuracy to conventional laboratory guides, in all directions except for vertical positioning.

Orthognathic and Temporomandibular Joint Surgery

Traditional orthognathic surgery consists of sequential steps, beginning with diagnostic impressions and mounted casts, cephalometric analysis, bite registrations,

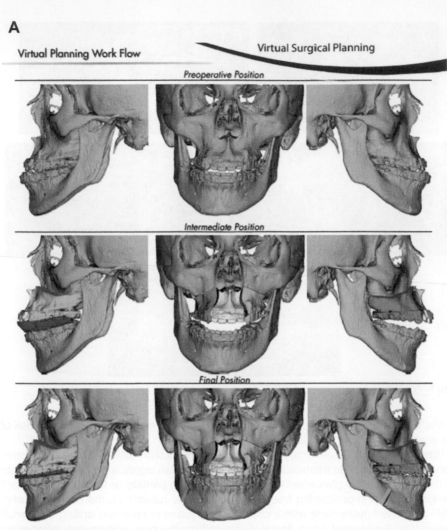

Fig. 10. (*A*) VSP using DICOM software to virtually plan a segmented LeFort I osteotomy with bilateral sagittal split osteotomy to correct facial asymmetry and occlusion. Conference calls are held with design engineers to discuss the planned movements for the surgical plan. This can be altered in all 3 dimensions and custom final splints can be fabricated to be used intraoperatively. (*B*) Intraoral photos of asymmetry and malocclusion. (*C*). VSP (3D Systems Medical Modeling in conjunction with KLS plating system) used to plan complete orthognathic surgery from the bony cuts to be replicated intraoperatively by using custom cutting jigs. This eliminates the need for an intermediate splint required to determine the final position of the maxilla in space. (*D*) Custom maxillary plates positioned into predetermined position, drastically decreasing the time it takes to bend plates intraoperatively. (*E*) Final occlusion with alignment of midlines and correction of asymmetry. (*Courtesy of* Edward Ellis, DDS, MS, San Antonio, TX.)

and model surgery with splint fabrication. Historically, it has been associated with extensive hours of preoperative planning and can be subject to critical errors. There are several disadvantages associated with traditional preoperative planning and model surgery. Some of these disadvantages include lack of time efficiency and the potential for error introduced with the initial steps, such as diagnostic impressions

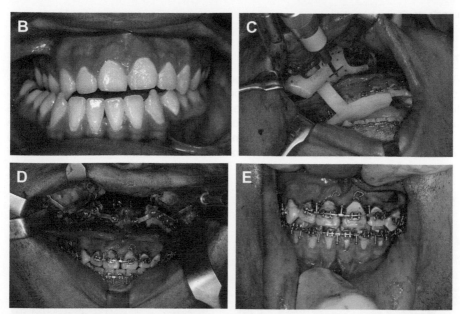

Fig. 10. (*continued*).

and cephalometric analysis. In addition, if the bite registration is inaccurate and does not appropriately reflect the patient's centric relation, this can lead to model surgery and splint fabrication that does not match the patient's anatomy.

Challenges encountered in orthognathic and TMJ surgery most commonly refer to the final occlusal position of the jaws. This is greatly influenced by the final positioning of the condyles in the glenoid fossa, as well as the 3D positioning of the jaws in space. Poor surgical planning; that is, incorrect registration of centric relation, can create undesired yaws or cants during surgery, which can result in suboptimal occlusal outcomes. These challenges can be partially overcome with the use of VSP software currently available. The process begins with obtaining a preoperative CBCT with the patient in centric relation. The CT dataset then gets converted into DICOM format, which can be used by several software programs to perform virtually simulated surgery. This allows the clinician the ability to perform simulated osteotomies and movements of the jaws in 3 dimensions (**Fig. 10**). It also offers the ability to fabricate custom interim and final splints, in addition to cutting jigs and custom plates to allow for splintless surgery (see **Fig. 10**).

In addition, a STL model can be created from the manipulated DICOM CT data of the patient, which can then be used to generate accurate, custom-fitted TMJ prostheses. VSP software allows the ability to not only perform surgical simulations and osteotomies on a computer but also allows accurate determination of the location and anatomy of important vital structures such as the inferior alveolar nerve. Finally, CAS software provides the ability to create custom cutting jigs used intraoperatively that eliminate the need for a surgical splint.

Advantages include improved ergonomics, decreased intraoperative time, and reduced duration of general anesthesia. Several studies have looked at the efficacy, accuracy, and time-reducing capabilities offered by CAS. A double-center clinical trial of 55 subjects found the accuracy to be within less than 1 mm between experimental and control groups.[1] A study by Xia and colleagues[12] has shown a statistically significant improvement in surgical outcomes of treatment of CMF deformities when comparing traditional model surgery with computer-simulated surgery.

Trauma and Facial Reconstruction

Reconstruction for traumatic facial injuries poses a great challenge to the oral and maxillofacial surgeon. CAS has been described for use in orbital, zygomaticocomplex, in addition to maxillary and mandibular injuries. Due to the anatomic complexity of the orbit, CAS offers the ability to presurgically compose custom orbital plates and to use intraoperative navigation to verify proper hardware placement (**Fig. 11**). Of particular importance is the ability of CAS to assist in adequate restoration of orbital anatomy and restoration of

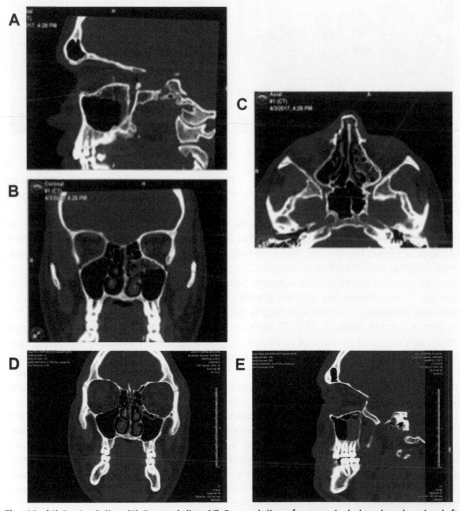

Fig. 11. (*A*) Sagittal slice. (*B*) Coronal slice. (*C*) Coronal slice of presurgical planning showing left orbital floor fracture. Green outline indicates unaffected side used to create the surgical virtual plan (*yellow outline*). (*D*) Coronal view. (*E*) Sagittal view. Postoperative CT scan of the left orbital reconstruction shown in Figs. 11-*D, E*. Accurate adaptation of plate to medial wall was achieved as predetermined by the virtual plan. Placement of the titanium plate in posterior orbit was shown to be in accurate, preplanned position to achieve optimal orbital volume restoration. This aspect of orbital reconstruction without computer assistance poses difficulty intraoperatively in the setting of decreased surgical access. In the final step, these postoperative CT images can be superimposed onto the virtual plan to confirm the accuracy of presurgical planning.

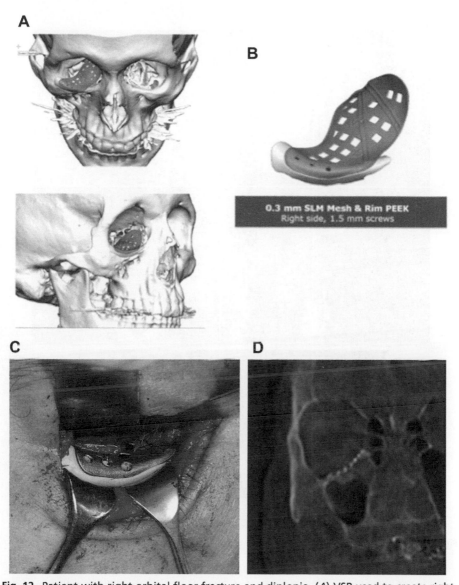

Fig. 12. Patient with right orbital floor fracture and diplopia. (*A*) VSP used to create right custom orbital plate for right orbital floor blowout fracture. (*B, C*) Virtually created custom orbital plate made of titanium with inferior polyether ether ketone (PEEK) component. (*D*) Intraoperative CT scanning used to confirm orbital fixation to identify any inaccuracies in the same operation. (*E*) Intraoperative navigation used to confirm the placement of the preplanned orbital plate. (*F*) Coronal (*left*) and sagittal (*right*) views of postoperative scan exemplifying accurate results and consistency with VSP. Intraoperative fusion navigation screenshot. CAD/CAM software is used to create a virtual plan for a left orbital floor reconstruction using the mirror image of the unaffected side (*green outline*). This can then be used intraoperatively with instrument tracking to ensure implanted hardware is fixated to the predetermined, most accurate achievable position.

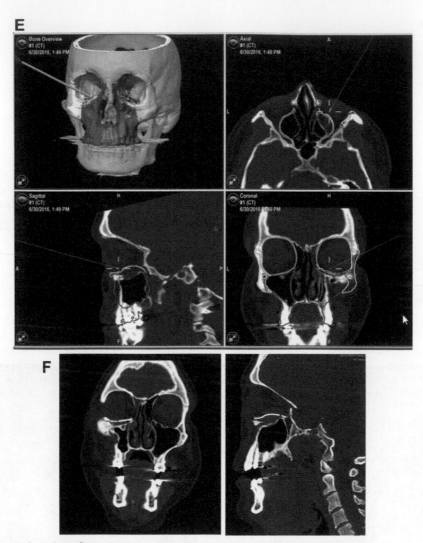

Fig. 12. (*continued*).

preinjury orbital volumes.[8] This is particularly important given the difficult nature involved in maintaining adequate globe projection and restoring orbital volume (**Fig. 12**).

The process begins with placement of an optical array on the patient's skull, which is kept stationary throughout the procedure. After the array has been positioned, the registration process begins with the selection of fiducial markers identified first on the virtual plan and then on the actual patient (see **Fig. 12**).[14]

Maxillomandibular Reconstruction

Computer-assisted planning and navigation has great utility in cases of tumor resection and facial reconstruction, as well as in TMJ reconstruction (**Fig. 13**). The patient's 3D data-set can be used to create a simulated surgical plan with identification of nearby structures and to locate necessary surgical margins required for ablation (**Fig. 14**). This information can later be used intraoperatively with a navigation system to ensure the preplanned margins are obtained while avoiding iatrogenic injury to adjacent vital structures.

In addition, the presurgical planning provides the capability to perform nerve mapping, which identifies the position and diameter of nerves. This information can be provided to nerve repair companies to preorder the predetermined size of nerve grafts that may need to be used intraoperatively in cases in which nerve lateralization and additional protection may be needed.

Other Applications

Although most of the use of CAS in CMF surgery and dentistry exist in reconstruction and implant placement, there are some other less common uses. For example, it is a challenge to obtain an excellent cosmetic result cases of cranial vault reconstruction. With CAS, the surgeon can use the patient's CT dataset to custom design a prosthetic calvarial implant, such as the polyether ether ketone (PEEK) implants. This can ensure accurate and esthetically satisfying results (**Fig. 15**).

DISCUSSION

Many advances have been made within the last 20 years regarding computer assistance to plan and navigate cases in dentistry and CMF surgery. Despite the recent advances, there are still some areas that can benefit from further advances in the technology. For instance, similar to the navigated dental implant handpiece, companies will be developing navigated drills in the near future to be used for CMF surgeries.

Although only a few, there are certain limitations to surgical navigation that can be the targets for further advances and improvements in the near future. For example, at this point, facial reconstruction is limited to unilateral cases due to the inability to mirror the unaffected side. This is a drawback to using surgical navigation for the

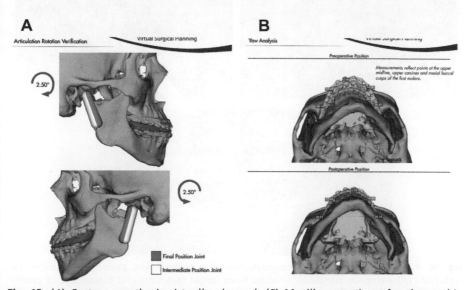

Fig. 13. (*A*) Custom prosthesis virtually planned. (*B*) Maxillary portion of orthognathic surgery can also be completed with the ability to correct for yaws and cants that may be difficult to do via traditional planning methods. (*Courtesy of* Daniel Perez, DDS, San Antonio, TX.)

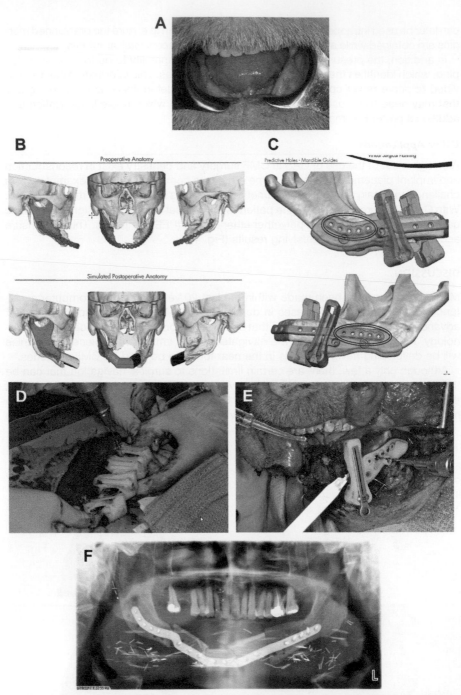

Fig. 14. A case of a mandibular reconstruction of a patient who underwent mandibular resection. (*A*) Atrophic mandible resulted from initial resection and placement of reconstruction plate. (*B, C*) VSP software used to plan mandibular reconstruction using virtual planning software. (*D, E*) Custom cutting jigs used intraoperatively to determine the precise location of the osteotomy sites. (*F*) Panoramic film of final mandibular hardware in place with precise adaptation and placement as preplanned with VSP.

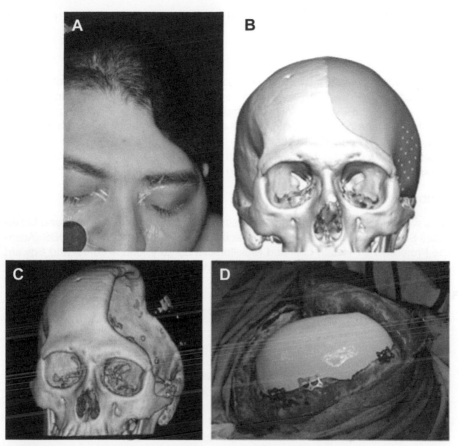

Fig. 15. (A) Left cranial defect after craniectomy. (B) 3D reconstructed image illustrating left cranial defect. (C) VSP with custom PEEK implant to reconstruct left cranial defect. (D). PEEK implant fixated in place with titanium plates and screws. (Courtesy of Ramesh Grandhi, MD, San Antonio, TX and Carlos G. Landaeta-Quinones, DDS, San Antonio, TX.)

planning of bilateral cases, such as for the excision of mandibular lesions and midface fractures.[9]

Some clinicians may argue that using CAS may expose the patient to increased radiation.[10] However, it may eliminate the need for additional radiographic imaging studies that are indicated if there is a doubt in the final surgical position. It is well-known that radiation doses for most CBCTs used to obtain the DICOM data are considered minimal. The following are estimated effective doses of common radiologic studies: single chest radiograph, 0.02 mSv; intraoral radiograph, 0.005 mSv; CT scan of the head, 2 mSv; CT scan of the neck, 4 mSv; CT scan of the chest, 8 mSv; and CT pulmonary embolism protocol, 15 mSv.[10]

However, with the accuracy that dynamic guided implant placement can be performed, the initial CBCT obtained for the initial planning seems minute. Block and colleagues[11] found significant differences in measurements comparing fully guided and partially guided navigation with freehand implant placement when using navigation. This saves the patient a visit and shortens the time it takes to complete restorative treatment plans. Within the near future, new technologies such as elastic fusion and augmented reality will be available in which reconstructions with a lack of references can be used.

SUMMARY

CAS has evolved over the past 20 years into advanced optical navigation systems with recent utility in CMF. Currently, CAS is most commonly used within CMF and dentistry for orthognathic and TMJ surgery, facial trauma, implantology, and maxillomandibular reconstruction. Despite the learning curve associated with using a new system, the technology adds increased accuracy and time efficiency to benefit patient surgical outcomes. In the near future, clinicians can look forward to further advancements in computer-assisted navigation and planning to further improve surgical outcomes.

ACKNOWLEDGMENTS

This work was supported by the University of Texas Department of Oral and Maxillofacial Surgery, San Antonio, Texas. Special thank you to Daniel Perez, DDS (Associate Professor, UT Health Oral and Maxillofacial Surgery, San Antonio) and Edward Ellis, III, MS, DDS (Chair, UT Health Oral and Maxillofacial Surgery, San Antonio).

REFERENCES

1. Hassfeld S, Mühling J. navigation in maxillofacial and craniofacial surgery. Computer aided surgery 1998;3(4):183–7.
2. Bell RB. Computer planning and intraoperative navigation in cranio-maxillofacial surgery. Oral Maxillofac Surg Clin North Am 2010;22:135–56.
3. Dai J, Wu J, Wang X, et al. An excellent navigation system and experience in craniomaxillofacial navigation surgery: a double-center study. Sci Rep 2016;6: 28242.
4. Nottmeier EW, Crosby TL. Timing of paired points and surface matching registration in three-dimensional (3D) image-guided spinal surgery. J Spinal Disord Tech 2007;20(4):268–70.
5. Block MS, Emery RW. Static or dynamic navigation for implant placement—choosing the method of guidance. J Oral Maxillofac Surg 2016;74:269–77.
6. Strong EB, Rafii A, Holhweg-Majert B, et al. Comparison of 3 optical navigation systems for computer-aided maxillofacial surgery. Arch Otolaryngol Head Neck Surg 2008;134(10):1080–4.
7. Gellrich N-C. Computer assisted oral and maxillofacial reconstruction. J Comput Inf Technology- CIT 14 2006;1:71–6.
8. Herford AS, Miller M, Lauritano F, et al. The use of virtual surgical planning and navigation in the treatment of orbital trauma. Chin J Traumatol 2017;20(1):9–13.
9. Azarmehr I, Stokbro K, Bell RB, et al. Surgical navigation: a systematic review of indications, treatments, and outcomes in oral and maxillofacial surgery. J Oral Maxillofac Surg 2017;75(9):1987–2005.
10. Bagheri S. Clinical review of oral and maxillofacial surgery. 2nd edition. A case-based approach. Mosby. 2013.
11. Block MS, Emery RW, Cullum DR, et al. Implant placement is more accurate using dynamic navigation. J Oral Maxillofac Surg 2017;75(7):1377–86.

Optical Coherence Tomography

Rujuta A. Katkar, BDS, MDS, MS[a],*, Satyashankara Aditya Tadinada, BDS, MDentSci[b],
Bennett T. Amaechi, BDS, MSc, PhD, MFDS RCPS (Glasg), FADI[c], Daniel Fried, PhD[d]

KEYWORDS

- Optical coherence tomography • Dental OCT • SS-OCT • PS-OCT

KEY POINTS

- Optical coherence tomography (OCT) is a noninvasive diagnostic technique providing cross-sectional images of biologic structures based on the differences in tissue optical properties.
- Different types of OCT including TD-OCT, FD-OCT, SS-OCT, PS-OCT are discussed.
- OCT has several potential applications in dentistry.
- The main limitations for clinical use of OCT in dentistry are high cost and lack of commercial availability.

OPTICAL COHERENCE TOMOGRAPHY

Optical coherence tomography (OCT) is a noninvasive diagnostic technique providing cross-sectional images of biologic structures based on the differences in tissue optical properties. It was first reported by Fujimoto and colleagues[1] in 1991. It is an interferometric technique that uses near-infrared (IR) light waves that reflect off the internal microstructure in a way that, in principle, is analogous to an ultrasonic pulse echo. It is possible to obtain real-time images with excellent axial resolution (<10 μm).[2] OCT has been widely used in numerous clinical applications, including gastroenterology, ophthalmology, and dermatology and is becoming popular as a promising technology in dentistry.

OPTICAL COHERENCE TOMOGRAPHY TYPES AND SPECIFICATIONS

OCT combines light from a low-coherence broadband light source with an interferometer to produce cross-sectional images of tissue structures generated as a result of

Disclosure: The authors have nothing to disclose.
[a] Department of Comprehensive Dentistry, UT Health, School of Dentistry, 7703 Floyd Curl Drive, San Antonio, TX 78229, USA; [b] Oral Health and Diagnostic Sciences, UConn Health, 263 Farmington Avenue, Farmington, CT 06030-1605, USA; [c] Department of Comprehensive Dentistry, University of Texas Health Science San Antonio, School of Dentistry, 7703 Floyd Curl Drive, San Antonio, TX 78229-3900, USA; [d] Department of Preventive and Restorative Dental Sciences, University of California, San Francisco, 707 Parnassus Avenue, San Francisco, CA 94143-0758, USA
* Corresponding author.
E-mail address: katkarr@uthscsa.edu

interaction between a partially coherent beam of optical radiation and tissue components.[1,3]

The early OCT systems were based on time-domain (TD) detection in which echo time delays of light were identified by measuring the interference signal as a function of time, while scanning the optical path length of the reference arm.[1,4] The light reflected from the sample and reference arms interferes within a Michelson or Mach-Zehnder interferometer. This interference signal is acquired by a photodiode or charge-coupled device that is dependent on the type of OCT. **Fig. 1** shows the first OCT type, TD-OCT. TD-OCT acquires various optical path lengths by moving a reference reflector.[5]

Another common type of OCT is the spectral domain OCT or Fourier domain (FD) OCT. A spectral domain OCT system is setup with almost the same components as TD-OCT but with an additional grating (for spatial Fourier transform), sensor array (usually charge-coupled device array), or spectrometer.[2] OCT has been revolutionized in recent years by the development of FD techniques that allow high-speed scanning without loss of sensitivity.[6] Swept-source (SS)-OCT is one of the implements of FD-OCT and uses a wavelength-tuned laser as the light source.[7] In SS-OCT, the spectrally resolved interference is derived from rapidly sweeping the wavelength of the laser. The high acquisition speed of SS-OCT, providing near real-time video-rate imaging while improving the overall signal-to-noise ratio of the acquired images, has made clinical applications of OCT more feasible.[8] In the authors'

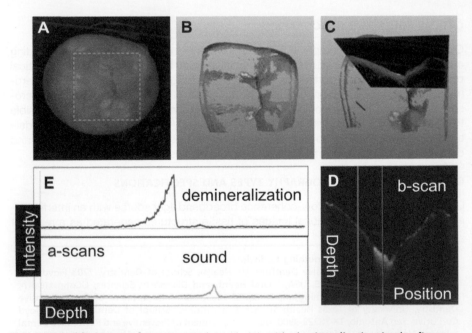

Fig. 1. A visible image of an extracted tooth (*A*) with demineralization in the fissure; a 5 × 5 mm box was cut to mark the region of interest. (*B, C*) Acquired CP-OCT three-dimensional scans segmented to show areas of demineralization (*red/yellow*). (*D*) A two-dimensional slice extracted from the image at the position indicated in *C* is shown. This is called a b-scan. The b-scan is displayed in grayscale with higher reflectivity in white corresponding to demineralization. (*E*) Two lineouts of depth versus intensity, called a-scans, were extracted (*red* and *blue lines*) at sound and lesion (demineralization) areas.

experience, TD-OCT loses signal-to-noise ratio at higher scanning speeds (>1 kHz), whereas FD-OCT systems do not. Therefore, FD-OCT is essential for clinical imaging particularly if three-dimensional (3D) images are to be acquired. However, it is misleading to claim that FD-OCT gives much better images than TD-OCT systems with greater penetration and resolution. One problem with FD methods is that half of the data points in an a-scan are lost when one does the Fourier transform, thus resulting in lower sampling.

OCT systems with appropriate broadband light sources usually demonstrate excellent axial resolution less than 20 μm. The transverse resolution is decided by the focus spot size on the sample. Higher transverse resolution may be achieved with a focused light.[2] Functional OCT, including Doppler OCT and polarization sensitive (PS-OCT), gathers more information in biologic tissues. Doppler OCT can provide the blood velocity and inflamed tissue volume information. However, PS-OCT can be used for structure orientation because of the polarization property.[2]

The high refractive indices of enamel and dentin result in high reflection at tooth surfaces that can mask the underlying tooth structure. PS-OCT is particularly valuable for imaging early caries lesions because the cross-polarization (CP) image can reduce the reflectivity from the tooth surface by orders of magnitude. In addition, the contrast between sound and demineralized enamel and dentin are higher in the CP image.[9] **Fig. 1** shows a 3D CP-OCT tomographic image of a $6 \times 6 \text{ mm}^2$ area of a tooth occlusal surface with demineralization in the fissure. The b-scan image shows position, depth, and the magnitude of the reflectivity or back-scattered light. Each pixel is displayed in a grayscale false color image with white indicating high reflectivity and black representing low reflectivity. Two a-scans of reflectivity versus depth are shown from sound and lesion areas. The reflectivity from the area of demineralization is orders of magnitude larger than the reflectivity from sound enamel.

Considering that the information collected cutting the object axially is obviously limited, it is more natural to see *en face* slices in the tissue in the way one sees them when looking through a microscope. Thus besides collecting a-scan (reflectivity vs depth graph) and longitudinal (b-scan), OCT has been demonstrated to produce a transverse or *en face* (c-scan) images.[10] Although an OCT b-scan image is produced either in the plane (x,z) or (y,z), a c-scan image is produced in the plane (x,y). Transverse images (c-scan) showed the *en face* slices of the tooth tissue like in confocal microscopy. Longitudinal images showed the depth of the lesion into the tooth tissue and the different structural layers of tooth tissue (enamel, dentin-enamel junction [DEJ], and dentin) in the same way as seen in ultrasound images. A-scans preformed in locations selected in the *en face* images can provide quantitative data about the reflectivity versus depth.[11,12] When in transversal regime, *en face* images collected at different depths are subsequently used to reconstruct 3D volumes of the tissue. The reconstruction allows software-inferred OCT longitudinal images at any transversal position in the stack. However, a-scan remains the best mode for quantitative analysis of the activity (demineralization or remineralization) of the caries lesion over time, and therefore could be exploited in the determination of the effect of caries therapeutic agents (eg, fluoride mouthrinse, fluoride dentifrice). Successive displays of transversal and longitudinal cuts at different positions in the 3D stack of *en face* OCT images give a direct view of the caries volume.

DENTAL OPTICAL COHERENCE TOMOGRAPHY

The first in vitro images of dental hard and soft tissue with OCT were acquired by Colston and colleagues in 1998.[13] Otis and colleagues[14] presented the first in vivo OCT images of human dental tissues with 12-μm axial resolution and 1310-nm center wavelength. They provided visual recording of the DEJ and periodontal structures. Feldchtein and colleagues[15] presented the first in vivo dental images and demonstrated that hard palate mucosa and gingiva mucosa could be visualized with OCT. Because the optical characteristics of the enamel and dentin differ because of structural and compositional factors, the two structures are distinguished from each other with the DEJ appearing as a dark borderline.[3] The early OCT studies focused mainly on the topics of dental soft and hard tissue morphology because of the limitation of system size and light source manufacture technology. With new developments in technology, OCT is now being applied in various fields in dentistry including dental caries, dental restorations (micro leakage), periodontal disease, tooth crack, and oral cancer (**Table 1**).[3,16]

Dental Caries

In OCT, tooth demineralization is distinguished from sound tissue based on the following two main principles: increased light scattering in porous demineralized tissue and depolarization of incident light by demineralized tissue. The latter necessitates PS-OCT or CP-OCT.[3] **Fig. 2** contains copolarization and CP images of demineralization in the fissure of the occlusal surface along with a matching transverse microradiograph and polarized light micrograph of a matching histologic section.[17] The contrast between the sound and demineralized enamel is much higher in the CP-OCT image. In addition the surface reflection is also much weaker in the CP-OCT image. The surface reflection is extremely strong for smooth surfaces. Enamel

Table 1	
Potential applications of OCT in dentistry	
Dental caries	Diagnosis of primary caries
	Diagnosis of recurrent/residual caries
	Extent of remineralization
	Integration with CAD/CAM technology for removal of caries and prosthesis fabrication
Dental restorations/ prostheses	Chair-side confirmation of the precision and accuracy of composite resin restorations
	Estimation of distance to the pulp while preparing the teeth with incorporation of OCT in a turbine, to avoid the risk of pulp exposure
	Evaluation of margins of Cr-Br prostheses
	Establishment of a non-destructive quality control system for predicting denture prosthesis treatment/repair
Endodontics	Diagnosis of tooth cracks
	Identification of pulp canals
Periodontal disease	Extent of alveolar bone loss
	Imaging and quantification of dental plaque
Dental implants	Localization of inferior alveolar canal and floor of maxillary sinus intraoperatively, avoiding accidental injuries during implant surgery
Soft tissue pathoses	Diagnosis of oral soft tissue disease with comparable results to pathologic diagnosis in near future (optical biopsy).
Dental education	Use of 3D constructed images based on OCT can be used in educational simulation systems.

Abbreviations: 3D, three-dimensional; CAD/CAM, computer-aided design/computer-aided manufacturing.

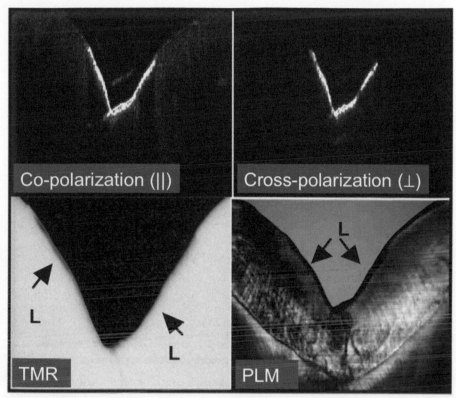

Fig. 2. Copolarization and cross-polarization PS-OCT b-scan images of a posterior tooth displayed in a false-color black-red-white intensity scale. A polarized light micrograph (PLM) and transverse microradiograph (TMR) of a matching tooth section are shown for comparison. (*From* Jones RS, Darling CL, Featherstone JDB, et al. Imaging artificial caries on the occlusal surfaces with polarization-sensitive optical coherence tomography. Caries Res 2006;40(2):85; with permission.)

and dentin are birefringent tissues so there is some reflectivity in the CP image from sound tissues. Several studies have shown that PS-OCT is suitable for early caries diagnosis to quantify lesion depth and mineral loss in the enamel or dentin.[18–21] The ability of PS-OCT to monitor remineralization and the formation of a distinct transparent surface zone has also been demonstrated in multiple studies.[22,23] **Fig. 3** shows PS-OCT copolarization and CP images of a bovine enamel sample with six windows showing sound, lesion, and lesion areas that have been exposed for 4, 8, and 12 days to a remineralization solution. There is minimal reflectivity in the sound regions outside the four windows, whereas the lesions have much higher contrast in the CP-OCT image. Although there was a high degree of remineralization, there was still incomplete remineralization of the body of the lesion. The most obvious change was the formation of a distinct transparent outer surface layer 50-μm thick. The depth of the lesion shown in **Fig. 3** was approximately 140 μm and the depth did not decrease after remineralization. The integrated reflectivity for this sample decreased by approximately 50% after 12 days, showing less reflectivity from the body of the lesion.[24] A 3D OCT image is obtained when a micromechanical system or galvanometer scanners are integrated with the OCT system.[25] 3D OCT systems have been used for several clinical

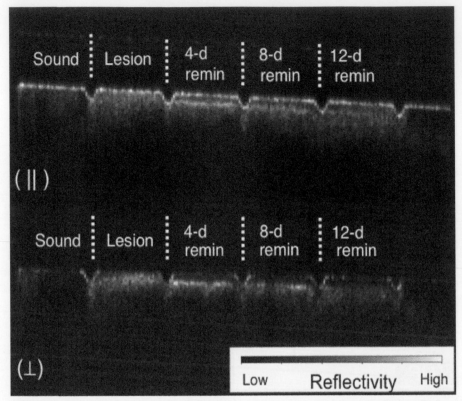

Fig. 3. PS-OCT b-scan images of a bovine enamel block showing the sound (protected) regions located on the extreme left and right side of the sample, the lesion area (0 days exposed to remin. soln) and the areas exposed for increasing periods of time to the remineralization solution, 4, 8, and 12 days. The double vertical line image represents the light reflected in the original polarization and the perpendicular image is the orthogonal polarization or cross-polarization image, which was used for analysis in these studies. The incisions are ~100 μm deep and separated by 1.4 mm. (*From* Kang H, Darling CL, Fried D. Nondestructive monitoring of the repair of enamel artificial lesions by an acidic remineralization model using polarization-sensitive optical coherence tomography. Dent Mater 2012;28(5):491; with permission.)

studies.[26–28] Images of a CP-SS-OCT are shown in **Fig. 4** along with a 3D image of demineralization that has developed next to an orthodontic bracket.[26]

Many clinicians are primarily interested in knowing how deep the occlusal lesions have actually penetrated into the tooth so that they can decide whether a restoration is necessary. Even though the optical penetration of near-IR light can easily exceed 7 mm through sound enamel to image lesions on proximal surfaces with high contrast, the large increase in light scattering caused by demineralization typically limits optical penetration in highly scattering lesions (also in dentin and bone) to 1 to 2 mm, thus cutting off the OCT signal before it reaches the DEJ.[29] Typically lesions spread laterally under the enamel on contacting the more soluble softer dentin. Therefore, OCT is used to determine if occlusal lesions have penetrated to the underlying dentin by detecting the lateral spread across the DEJ. In a clinical study, 12 out of 14 of the lesions examined in vivo using OCT exhibited increased reflectivity below the DEJ indicating that the lesions had spread to the dentin.[30] Because none of the lesions showed

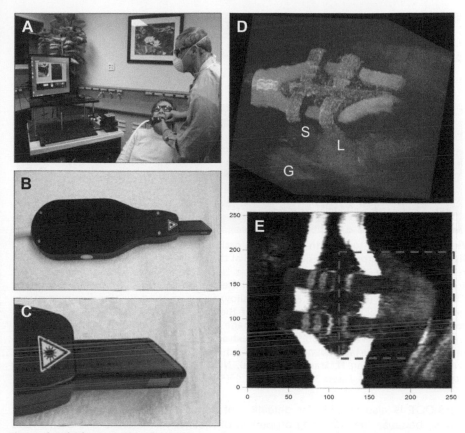

Fig. 4. (*A–C*) Photographs of a volunteer being scanned with a 3D CP-OCT system, along with close-up views of the scanning handpiece and the 6 × 6 mm scanning window at the end of the scanner. (*D*) Surface rendering of 6 × 6 × 7 mm 3D CP-OCT image. G, gingiva; L, lesion; S, sound. (*E*) Collapsed two-dimensional image of ΔR (rotated by 90°) showing the area monitored over time in *red box*. (*Adapted from* Nee A, Chan K, Kang H, et al. Longitudinal monitoring of demineralization peripheral to orthodontic brackets using cross polarization optical coherence tomography. J Dent 2014;42(5):547–55; with permission.)

up on a radiograph, this demonstrates a remarkable improvement over existing technology.[30,31] The same approach can be used to detect approximal lesions from the occlusal surface.[32,33] This is demonstrated in **Fig. 5** using 3D CP-OCT and near-IR reflectance and occlusal transillumination. The depth of the lesion below the occlusal surface is clearly shown.[28]

Even though the penetration depth of near-IR light is more limited in dentin than for enamel, one can still acquire images of early root caries and demineralization in dentin.[34] PS-OCT studies have successfully measured demineralization in simulated caries models in dentin and on root surfaces (cementum).[18,25,35] PS-OCT can effectively be used to discriminate demineralized dentin from sound dentin and cementum.[18] PS-OCT has also been used to measure remineralization on dentin surfaces and to detect the formation of a highly mineralized layer on the lesion surface after exposure to a remineralization solution.[25] OCT has also been used to help discriminate between noncarious cervical lesions and root caries in vivo.[36]

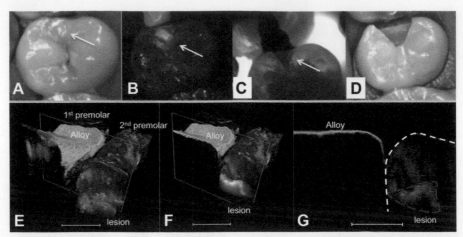

Fig. 5. Images of a tooth with a suspected occlusal lesion in the central fissure (stained fissure) and an interproximal lesion indicated at the position of the *arrow* in the visible light reflectance image (*A*) of the tooth are shown. Near-IR reflectance (*B*) and near-IR occlusal transillumination images (*C*). Visible image of the preparation (*D*) is also shown. A rendered CP-OCT 3D image (*E*) shows the amalgam (alloy) filling on the adjoining first premolar in *green* and the lesion in *red*. The length of the bar in images (*E–G*) is 300 μm. (*F*) The same 3D CP-OCT image is shown with the image truncated at the position of the extracted b-scan to better show the lesion. (*G*) In the extracted b-scan the surface of the second premolar and the subsurface lesion are shown by the *white* and *red dashed lines*, respectively. (*From* Simon JC, Kang H, Staninec M, et al. Near-IR and CP-OCT imaging of suspected occlusal caries lesions. Lasers Surg Med 2017;49(3):222; with permission.)

PS-OCT is also suitable for detection of caries around restoration (secondary caries), because the scattering properties of restorative materials and dental hard tissue have marked differences.[21] However, Lenton and colleagues[37] tried to use CP-OCT to assess the presence of secondary caries at subsurface composite restorations.

Because most OCT images obtained from the occlusal surfaces could not clearly display the pulp chamber within the tooth, and it was impossible to observe the distance of the caries from the dental pulp, radiographic examination is still considered to be necessary in cases exhibiting significant irreversible pulpitis symptoms.[33,38] However, OCT can display the location of the pulp beneath the cavity floor during the deep preparation to avoid pulpal exposure.[39–41] Iino and colleagues[42] found that OCT could image the location of the second mesiobuccal canal in maxillary molars in vitro, hence its potential use for endodontic treatment. *En face* (c-scan) OCT imaging has the potential to be helpful in this aspect.

Microleakage/Detection of Gap Formation and Secondary Caries at Tooth-Restoration Interface

Dental radiographs are frequently used in the clinic to detect a radiolucent zone that is associated with the presence of a thick adhesive layer, secondary caries, or a gap. However, loss of the interfacial seal appears undetectable by conventional dental radiographs because the size of these gaps has been reported to range from 0.3 to 16 μm.[43] This is readily viewed on OCT images as a clear line of increase in the signal intensity and is used for rapid detection of gaps at the restoration interface.[44,45] However, accurate quantification of these gaps depends on the angulation of the incident laser beam.[46] In addition to visualization of gaps at the interface, OCT imaging can also detect voids or air bubbles of different sizes within the composite restoration.[47,48]

Tooth Fracture/Crack

Shemesh and colleagues[49] presented the first work on the use of OCT to image cracks in teeth using an OCT probe that is placed in a root canal. Tooth fractures are categorized into five major classes: craze line, fractured cusp, cracked tooth, split tooth, and vertical root fracture.[50] Craze line is the initial tooth crack, and asymptomatic itself, which occurs in the enamel surface parallel to the prismatic orientation by occlusal forces or thermocycling. A cracked tooth is defined as a crack extending from the occlusal surface of the tooth apically without separation of the two segments.[50] Detection of tooth crack has been a diagnostic challenge and current methods, such as radiography, transillumination, methylene blue dyes, and operative microscopic examination, have their own limitations. SS-OCT has shown superior results compared with transillumination for detection of naturally formed enamel cracks and whole-thickness enamel cracks in vitro, with significantly higher reproducibility among three observers.[51] Cracks extending beyond the DEJ can also be imaged through OCT, thus aiding determination of the crack penetration depth. SS-OCT could detect vertical root fractures of extracted human teeth.[52] However, the current SS-OCT setup cannot be used for detecting root fractures at the subgingival zone through an open root canal because of the probe design and through the gingiva because of signal attenuation in the soft tissue and bone. Application of SS-OCT for tooth fracture detection is limited to the coronal portion in which laser light is irradiated.[51,53] Further development of technology, such as systems with improved transmission into soft tissue and special imaging probes for detection of the subgingival zone, can improve the diagnostic accuracy for detecting a tooth fracture and enhance the demands of OCT for clinical use.[54]

Periodontal Diseases

OCT has been used in vitro and in vivo in animal models for demonstration of periodontal tissues and subgingival calculus. The enamel-cementum and the gingiva-tooth interfaces can be clearly visualized, indicating OCT is a potentially useful technique for diagnosis of periodontal diseases. In addition, imaging and quantification of dental plaque biofilm using CP-OCT has also been demonstrated.[55–58]

Oral Cancer

Studies have shown that OCT could detect neoplasia-related epithelial and subepithelial changes throughout carcinogenesis (**Fig. 6**). In a study done by Campos and Hugo,[59] a test group of 39 mice was treated with nitroquinoline 1-oxide (4NQO) to chemically induce malignant mucosal lesions on the tongue; an additional 10 mice served as the untreated control group for this study. The posterior region of the tongue where malignant transformation was induced was evaluated with the use of OCT and histopathologic analyses. In this study, recognition of normal tissue architecture was good between the two modalities but ability to discern between zones of normal and malignant transformation was not overwhelming. Although the technique for analyzing the areas of interest using histologic staining is fairly standardized, OCT does not have established protocols, which are currently being researched. This proof of concept study shows that normal and malignant transformation can be evaluated in vivo without actually needing to extract a piece of the tissue for analysis. This area has significant promise; it can possibly be solved by constructing probes with superior engineering designing, establishing scanning protocols, and by developing post-processing algorithms to help early detection.

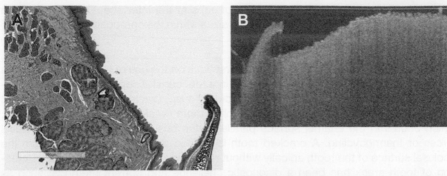

Fig. 6. Histologic image (hematoxylin-eosin, original magnification ×4) (*A*) and OCT image (*B*) of the posterior aspect of a mouse tongue with hyperkeratosis.

Tissue Characterization and Quantification of Optical Density

OCT is broadly considered analogous to ultrasound imaging with the sound component substituted with light. Just as different tissues resonate to sound differently, different tissues also reflect light differently based on their tissue density, texture, and property (**Fig. 7**). With evolution of OCT tissue characterization based on optical density has become possible. One good way to do this is to have known tissues with uniform density distribution, obtain an optical density value, and correlate those values to established density numbers from computed tomography or cone beam computed tomography images.[60] Because there is no standardization of OCT engines or the wavelengths at this point, multiple machine-specific look-up tables are being used for tissue quantification.

Machine Learning Using Optical Coherence Tomography Images

Most imaging modalities produce images as a balance between signal and noise. To date signal-to-noise ratios have only been evaluated in the discernible range to the

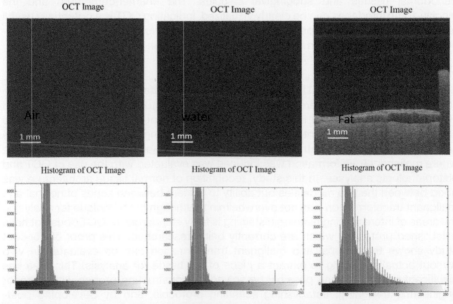

Fig. 7. OCT images and post-processed histogram images of the same tissues.

human eye. With the development of advanced computer systems, significant memory storage and pattern recognition capabilities arranged in compact microchips is available to the end users. Along those lines, a new concept called machine learning is helping glean valuable information from what would have been previously considered noise. Once certain known processes, such as mineralization patterns or tissue transformations, are understood and quantified by the user, neural networks learn the patterns and self-teach themselves in picking up the minutest of changes thus giving the clinician the ability to decide if such changes trigger the necessity for further investigation and or intervention. Images generated by OCT can now be post-processed using advanced algorithms to assign a meaningful representation to otherwise undiscernible noise.[61] The future is definitely going to be about fusion imaging and postprocessing and OCT will play a significant role in that endeavor.

LIMITATIONS FOR CLINICAL USE OF OPTICAL COHERENCE TOMOGRAPHY IN DENTISTRY AND FUTURE PERSPECTIVES FROM LATEST RESEARCH

Principal issues are cost and lack of commercial availability. Because of the high cost of the component parts, OCT machines are costly when produced for commercialization. This high cost limits sales and discourages manufacturers. Future research should be directed toward the following:

1. Increasing the optical penetration of OCT to permit accurate diagnosis of proximal caries lesions, lesions underneath and around restorations, and more deeply located occlusal caries.
2. Developing imaging software and algorithms for image analysis, contrast measurement, and image registration for real-time simultaneous processing and analysis of images.
3. Increasing the contrast between sound and carious tissues.

REFERENCES

1. Huang D, Swanson EA, Lin CP, et al. Optical coherence tomography. Science 1991;254(5035):1178–81.
2. Hsieh YS, Ho YC, Lee SY, et al. Dental optical coherence tomography. Sensors (Basel) 2013;13(7):8928–49.
3. Shimada Y, Sadr A, Sumi Y, et al. Application of optical coherence tomography (OCT) for diagnosis of caries, cracks, and defects of restorations. Curr Oral Health Rep 2015;2(2):73–80.
4. Fujimoto JG, DW. Introduction to optical coherence tomography. In: Drexler W, FJ, editors. Optical coherence tomography. Springer; 2008. 1-2-45.
5. Schmitt JM. Optical coherence tomography (OCT): a review. IEEE J Sel Top Quantum Electron 1999;5(4):1205–15.
6. Leitgeb R, Hitzenberger CK, Fercher AF. Performance of Fourier domain vs. time domain optical coherence tomography. Opt Express 2003;11(8):889–94.
7. Chinn S, Swanson E, Fujimoto J. Optical coherence tomography using a frequency-tunable optical source. Opt Lett 1997;22(5):340–2.
8. Choma MA, Sarunic MV, Yang C, et al. Sensitivity advantage of swept source and Fourier domain optical coherence tomography. Opt Express 2003;11(18):2183–9.
9. Fried D, Xie J, Shafi S, et al. Imaging caries lesions and lesion progression with polarization sensitive optical coherence tomography. J Biomed Opt 2002;7(4):618–27.

10. Podoleanu AG, Seeger M, Dobre GM, et al. Transversal and longitudinal images from the retina of the living eye using low coherence reflectometry. J Biomed Opt 1998;3(1):12–20.

11. Amaechi BT, Higham SM, Podoleanu AG, et al. Use of optical coherence tomography for assessment of dental caries: quantitative procedure. J Oral Rehabil 2001;28(12):1092–3.

12. Amaechi BT, Podoleanu AG, Komarov GN, et al. Application of optical coherence tomography for imaging and assessment of early dental caries lesions. Laser Phys 2003;13(5):703–10.

13. Colston BW, Sathyam US, DaSilva LB, et al. Dental OCT. Opt Express 1998;3(6):230–8.

14. Otis LL, Everett MJ, Sathyam US, et al. Optical coherence tomography: a new imaging: technology for dentistry. J Am Dent Assoc 2000;131(4):511–4.

15. Feldchtein F, Iksanov R, Gelikonov G, et al. In vivo OCT imaging of hard and soft tissue of the oral cavity. Opt Express 1998;3(6):239–50.

16. Ding J, Ebihara A, Watanabe S, et al. Application of Optical Coherence Tomography to Identify Pulp Exposure During Access Cavity Preparation Using an Er:YAG Laser. Photomedicine and Laser Surgery 2014;32(6):356–9.

17. Jones RS, Darling CL, Featherstone JDB, et al. Imaging artificial caries on the occlusal surfaces with polarization-sensitive optical coherence tomography. Caries Res 2006;40(2):81–9.

18. Lee C, Darling CL, Fried D. Polarization-sensitive optical coherence tomographic imaging of artificial demineralization on exposed surfaces of tooth roots. Dent Mater 2009;25(6):721–8.

19. Chen Y, Otis L, Piao D, et al. Characterization of dentin, enamel, and carious lesions by a polarization-sensitive optical coherence tomography system. Appl Opt 2005;44(11):2041–8.

20. Louie T, Lee C, Hsu D, et al. Clinical assessment of early tooth demineralization using polarization sensitive optical coherence tomography. Lasers Surg Med 2010;42(10):898–905.

21. Baumgartner A, Dichtl S, Hitzenberger CK, et al. Polarization-sensitive optical coherence tomography of dental structures. Caries Res 2000;34(1):59–69.

22. Jones RS, Fried D. Remineralization of enamel caries can decrease optical reflectivity. J Dent Res 2006;85(9):804–8.

23. Jones RS, Darling CL, Featherstone JDB, et al. Remineralization of in vitro dental caries assessed with polarization-sensitive optical coherence tomography. J Biomed Opt 2006;11(1):014016.

24. Lee RC, Kang H, Darling CL, et al. Automated assessment of the remineralization of artificial enamel lesions with polarization-sensitive optical coherence tomography. Biomed Opt Express 2014;5(9):2950.

25. Manesh SK, Darling CL, Fried D. Polarization-sensitive optical coherence tomography for the nondestructive assessment of the remineralization of dentin. J Biomed Opt 2009;14(4):044002.

26. Nee A, Chan K, Kang H, et al. Longitudinal monitoring of demineralization peripheral to orthodontic brackets using cross polarization optical coherence tomography. J Dent 2014;42(5):547.

27. Chan KH, Tom H, Lee RC, et al. Clinical monitoring of smooth surface enamel lesions using CP-OCT during nonsurgical intervention. Lasers Surg Med 2016;48(10):915–23.

28. Simon JC, Kang H, Staninec M, et al. Near-IR and CP-OCT imaging of suspected occlusal caries lesions. Lasers Surg Med 2017;49(3):215–24.

29. Darling CL, Huynh GD, Fried D. Light scattering properties of natural and artificially demineralized dental enamel at 1310 nm. J Biomed Opt 2006;11(3):34023.
30. Douglas SM, Fried D, Darling CL. Imaging natural occlusal caries lesions with optical coherence tomography. Proc SPIE Int Soc Opt Eng 2010; 7549:75490N.
31. Staninec M, Douglas SM, Darling CL, et al. Non-destructive clinical assessment of occlusal caries lesions using near-IR imaging methods. Lasers Surg Med 2011;43(10):951–9.
32. Ngaotheppitak P, Darling CL, Fried D, et al. PS-OCT of occlusal and interproximal caries lesions viewed from occlusal surfaces. Lasers in Dentistry XII 6137(L),1-9 (2006).
33. Shimada Y, Nakagawa H, Sadr A, et al. Noninvasive cross-sectional imaging of proximal caries using swept-source optical coherence tomography (SS-OCT) in vivo. J Biophotonics 2014;7(7):506–13.
34. Amaechi BT, Podoleanu AG, Komarov G, et al. Quantification of root caries using optical coherence tomography and microradiography: a correlational study. Oral Health Prev Dent 2004;2(4):377–82.
35. Manesh SK, Darling CL, Fried D. Nondestructive assessment of dentin demineralization using polarization-sensitive optical coherence tomography after exposure to fluoride and laser irradiation. J Biomed Mater Res B Appl Biomater 2009;90(2):802–12.
36. Wada I, Shimada Y, Ikeda M, et al. Clinical assessment of non carious cervical lesion using swept-source optical coherence tomography. J Biophotonics 2015; 8(10):846–54.
37. Lenton P, Rudney J, Chen R, et al. Imaging in vivo secondary caries and ex vivo dental biofilms using cross-polarization optical coherence tomography. Dent Mater 2012;28(7):792–800.
38. Shimada Y, Sadr A, Burrow MF, et al. Validation of swept-source optical coherence tomography (SS-OCT) for the diagnosis of occlusal caries. J Dent 2010; 38(8):655–65.
39. Braz AK, Kyotoku BB, Gomes AS. In vitro tomographic image of human pulp-dentin complex: optical coherence tomography and histology. J Endod 2009; 35(9):1218–21.
40. Kyotoku BB, Maia AM, Gomes AS. In vitro imaging of remaining dentin and pulp chamber by optical coherence tomography: comparison between 850 and 1280nm. J Biomed Opt 2009;14(2):024009.
41. Fujita R, Komada W, Nozaki K, et al. Measurement of the remaining dentin thickness using optical coherence tomography for crown preparation. Dent Mater J 2014;33(3):355–62.
42. Iino Y, Ebihara A, Yoshioka T, et al. Detection of a second mesiobuccal canal in maxillary molars by swept-source optical coherence tomography. J Endod 2014;40(11):1865–8.
43. Sun J, Eidelman N, Lin-Gibson S. 3D mapping of polymerization shrinkage using X-ray micro-computed tomography to predict microleakage. Dent Mater 2009; 25(3):314–20.
44. Makishi P, Shimada Y, Sadr A, et al. Non-destructive 3D imaging of composite restorations using optical coherence tomography: marginal adaptation of self-etch adhesives. J Dent 2011;39(4):316–25.
45. Bakhsh TA, Sadr A, Shimada Y, et al. Non-invasive quantification of resin–dentin interfacial gaps using optical coherence tomography: validation against confocal microscopy. Dent Mater 2011;27(9):915–25.

46. Park K, Schneider H, Haak R. Assessment of interfacial defects at composite restorations by swept source optical coherence tomography. J Biomed Opt 2013; 18(7):076018.

47. Nazari A, Sadr A, Shimada Y, et al. 3D assessment of void and gap formation in flowable resin composites using optical coherence tomography. J Adhes Dent 2013;15(3):237–43.

48. Shimada Y, Sadr A, Nazari A, et al. 3D evaluation of composite resin restoration at practical training using swept-source optical coherence tomography (SS-OCT). Dent Mater J 2012;31(3):409–17.

49. Shemesh H, van Soest G, Wu M, et al. Basic research—technology: diagnosis of vertical root fractures with optical coherence tomography. J Endod 2008;34: 739–42.

50. Rivera E, Walton R. Cracking the cracked tooth code: detection and treatment of various longitudinal tooth fractures. ENDODONTICS: colleagues for excellence newsletter. 2008.

51. Imai K, Shimada Y, Sadr A, et al. Noninvasive cross-sectional visualization of enamel cracks by optical coherence tomography in vitro. J Endod 2012;38(9): 1269–74.

52. Yoshioka T, Sakaue H, Ishimura H, et al. Detection of root surface fractures with swept-source optical coherence tomography (SS-OCT). Photomed Laser Surg 2013;31(1):23–7.

53. Fried WA, Simon JC, Lucas S, et al. Near-IR imaging of cracks in teeth. Proc SPIE Int Soc Opt Eng 2014;8929:89290Q.

54. Shokri A, Khajeh S. In vitro comparison of the effect of different slice thicknesses on the accuracy of linear measurements on cone beam computed tomography images in implant sites. J Craniofac Surg 2015;26(1):157–60.

55. Colston BW Jr, Everett MJ, Da Silva LB, et al. Imaging of hard- and soft-tissue structure in the oral cavity by optical coherence tomography. Appl Opt 1998; 37(16):3582–5.

56. Baek JH, Na J, Lee BH, et al. Optical approach to the periodontal ligament under orthodontic tooth movement: a preliminary study with optical coherence tomography. Am J Orthod Dentofacial Orthop 2009;135(2):252–9.

57. Hsieh Y, Ho Y, Lee S, et al. Subgingival calculus imaging based on swept-source optical coherence tomography. J Biomed Opt 2011;16(7):071409.

58. Chen R, Rudney J, Aparicio C, et al. Quantifying dental biofilm growth using cross-polarization optical coherence tomography. Letters in Applied Microbiology 2012; 54(6):537–42.

59. Campos J, Hugo C. Efficacy of optical coherence tomography in the detection of potentially malignant oral mucosal lesions of the tongue: an animal model. Master's Theses. 2014. 666. Available at: https://opencommons.uconn.edu/gs_theses/666. Accessed April 10, 2018.

60. Mahdian M, Salehi HS, Lurie AG, et al. Tissue characterization using optical coherence tomography and cone beam computed tomography: a comparative pilot study. Oral Surg Oral Med Oral Pathol Oral Radiol 2016;122(1):98–108.

61. Karimian N, Salehi HS, Mahdian M, et al. Deep learning classifier with optical coherence tomography images for early dental caries detection. Proc. SPIE BiOS 10473, Lasers in Dentistry XXIV, 1047304. San Francisco, California, February 8, 2018.

Fluorescence and Near-Infrared Light Transillumination

Bennett T. Amaechi, BDS, MSc, PhD, MFDS RCPS (Glasg), FADI[a],*,
Adepitan A. Owosho, BChD[b,c], Daniel Fried, PhD[d]

KEYWORDS

- Autofluorescence • Near infra-red transillumination • Early detection • Dental caries
- Oral cancer • Osteoradionecrosis • Optical devices • Fluorescence technologies

KEY POINTS

- Technologies using autofluorescence of tooth and red fluorescence of bacterial metabolites for visualization and quantitative analysis of both early caries and dental plaque were discussed.
- Fluorescence-guided surgery, using devices with fluorescent light filters, aids surgeons in applying bone-preserving operative principles during surgical management of patients with osteoradionecrosis and medication-related osteonecrosis of the jaw.
- Autofluorescence devices aid in evaluation of oral mucosa for identification of premalignant and malignant lesions, and identifying the appropriate margin for tumor resection.
- The potential of novel imaging configurations such as near-infrared light reflectance and transillumination for imaging caries lesions on both proximal and occlusal surfaces of teeth were discussed.
- Evidence-based clinical practice guideline and most literature reviews recommend these diagnostic devices to be used only as adjuncts to clinical decision making.

The early detection and clinical staging of the presence, activity, and severity of a disease is of paramount importance in the deployment of treatment strategies that use either nonsurgical modalities or tissue-preserving surgical principles. Hence, it is generally recognized that the development of new technologies for the detection of

Disclosure: The authors have nothing to disclose.
[a] Department of Comprehensive Dentistry, School of Dentistry, University of Texas Health Science Center at San Antonio, 7703 Floyd Curl Drive, San Antonio, TX 78229-3900, USA;
[b] Department of Oral and Maxillofacial Pathology, College of Dental Medicine, University of New England, Goddard Hall, Room 212, 716 Stevens Avenue, Portland, ME 04103, USA;
[c] Oral Medicine, College of Dental Medicine, University of New England, Goddard Hall, Room 212, 716 Stevens Avenue, Portland, ME 04103, USA; [d] Division of Biomaterials and Bioengineering, Department of Preventive and Restorative Dental Sciences, University of California, San Francisco, 707 Parnassus Avenue, San Francisco, CA 94143-0758, USA
* Corresponding author.
E-mail address: amaechi@uthscsa.edu

any disease at an early stage of its formation could provide health and economic benefits, ranging from timely preventive interventions to decreased costs of surgical treatment. Thus, a variety of innovative technologies have been developed and introduced in the past few years to aid clinicians not only in early oral disease detection, but to make a firm diagnosis and treat cases conservatively. This article describes the various technologies based on either autofluorescence of body tissue or near-infrared (NIR) light illumination, tailored to aid practitioners in detecting and quantitatively monitoring oral diseases such as dental caries and oral cancer at the earliest stage of their formation, or in conservative surgical excision of necrotic bones in diseases such as chronic osteomyelitis, osteoradionecrosis (ORN), and medication-related osteonecrosis of the jaw (MRONJ). The current applications of these technologies are also discussed. The data discussed are primarily based on published scientific studies and reviews from case reports, clinical trials, and in vitro and in vivo studies. References have been traced manually, by MEDLINE, or through manufacturer's websites. Although some of the devices are fully developed and commercially available, others are still under development. The devices vary in their modes of action as well as their capability as diagnostic aids.

THE FLUORESCENCE SYSTEMS

Technologies based on autofluorescence use the alteration in natural fluorescence of a body tissue when the tissue becomes diseased to discriminate between a diseased tissue and the surrounding sound tissue.[1-9] Based on this principle, many technologies have been developed and introduced for clinical diagnosis of dental caries and oral cancer, surgical excision of necrotic bone tissues, and quantification of dental plaque.[1,8-19] However, evidence-based clinical practice guideline and most literature reviews recommend these fluorescence-based diagnostic devices to be used only as adjuncts to clinical decision making.[20-22] Particularly with the devices tailored for caries diagnosis, the output from these technologies should rarely be used to recommend surgical intervention considering the significant consequences of a false-positive or false-negative detection and diagnosis. In caries management, the inability of these devices to differentiate whether a suspected lesion is a stain, an arrested lesion, or hypomineralization precludes the use of these systems for intervention decisions. The applications of the fluorescence-based technologies in various aspects of oral disease management are discussed herein.

Application of Tissue Autofluorescence Systems in Caries Management

Fluorescence-based systems have been developed and introduced for clinical assessment, diagnosis, and monitoring of dental caries on the accessible tooth surfaces (occlusal, buccal, and lingual). These systems operate on the principle that sound tooth structure fluoresces with a distinct green color when illuminated with a specific spectrum of violet-blue light.[1] However, when the tooth enamel is demineralized (a caries lesion), the observed autofluorescence of a tooth is decreased owing to increased scattering of the incident light (**Fig. 1**).[1-3] The distribution of the green-emitting fluorophores is higher for dentin than for enamel and greatest at the dentin–enamel junction. An increase in scattering coefficient implies a decrease in mean free photon path length and hence the chance of a photon being absorbed by a fluorophore and a fluorescent photon being emitted is lowered. Where demineralization (a caries lesion) exists, the light travels shorter distances into the tooth, and the view on the dentin–enamel junction is blocked. As a result, we see a dark spot of

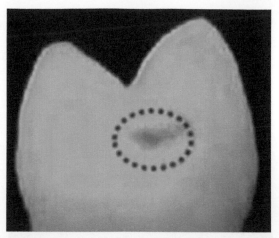

Fig. 1. When a tooth surface is viewed with a fluorescence-based system, early caries lesions appear as dark spots on a green background of healthy enamel. Fluorescence-based systems rely on contrast differences between sound and demineralized enamel for visual enhancement of caries lesions, making them very sensitive. (*Courtesy of* Inspektor Research Systems BV, Bussum, Netherlands.)

reduced fluorescence surrounded by bright green fluorescence from the sound tooth areas.[13] Fluorescence-based devices tailored for caries detection rely on this contrast between sound and demineralized enamel for the visual enhancement of caries detection. Contrast differences are much greater than when the teeth are viewed under normal white light conditions.[10] The reduction in autofluorescence owing to demineralization has been shown with some devices to correlate well with actual mineral loss, and can be quantified with proprietary software as an indirect measure of enamel porosity or caries lesion.[11,12]

The fluorescence-based systems possess several potential benefits as follows.

- The excitation light used in these systems is white light and of relatively low intensity; thus, examination presents no danger to patient or operator.
- The fluorescence-based systems possess high sensitivity owing to the high contrast between the sound and demineralized tissues. This gives these systems the potential for (a) easier and faster caries lesion detection, and (b) detection of the earliest stage of lesion development (see **Fig. 1**).[10,12,20] However, the specificity of these devices tend to be low considering that they detect stains and developmental hypomineralization, such as fluorosis, as caries lesions.[1–5,10–12,23–29]
- Currently existing fluorescence-based caries detection devices permit the quantitative documentation of the changing activities (progression, arrest, or reversed) of the lesion during treatment, and as such can monitor lesion activities over time, if confounding factors are well-controlled to maintain reliability (**Fig. 2**). However, most available systems do not have independent longitudinal studies supporting this type of application; thus, the sensitivity, specificity, accuracy, and reliability of most of these devices in performing this function may not meet acceptable expectation.[20]
- Most fluorescence-based devices are able to show digital images of the tooth surface and the associated lesions, thus, facilitating patient education and motivation with digitized images of the caries lesion (see **Fig. 1**).

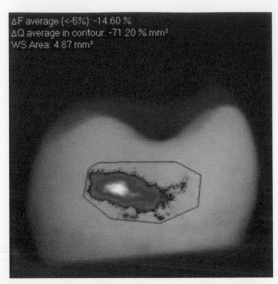

ΔF average (<-5%): -14.60 %
ΔQ average in contour: -71.20 %.mm²
WS Area: 4.87 mm²

Fig. 2. Some fluorescence-based systems use software programs to automatically give values for percentage of fluorescence radiance loss (ΔF [%]), lesion area (mm²), and volume of demineralization (ΔQ [%.mm²]). ΔQ is the unit for monitoring demineralization and remineralization. The varying colors represent varying levels of demineralization.

However, the fluorescence-based systems have some drawbacks that lower their accuracy and reliability for use as a sole diagnostic tool for dental caries management.

- Fluorescence-based systems cannot distinguish between stained and demineralized surfaces, and this factor grossly biases its use on the occlusal pits and fissures that commonly bear stains. Furthermore, staining of the lesion exaggerates fluorescence loss, portraying further demineralization when the lesion is actually remineralizing or arrested.[10] Thus, the fluorescence-based systems demonstrate the least validity, specificity, and reliability in occlusal pits/fissures where they are most needed.
- Both early caries lesions and development hypomineralization present clinically as white spot lesions; thus, clinicians need devices that can distinguish these 2 types of lesions. However, when viewed with the fluorescence systems, both lesions present as dark spots and cannot accurately be distinguished by these systems, which further precludes the use of these systems for intervention decisions.
- The contrast between carious and sound enamel may be masked by moisture on the tooth surface. Thus, these devices can only be reliable and accurate for monitoring lesion change over time if a standardized drying method, to maintain the same level of lesion hydration at each examination, is used; however, this step has not been taken in any longitudinal trial using these devices.[2,12,20]
- The fluorescence systems cannot indicate the depth of the caries lesion to aid the clinician in decision on treatment strategy; thus, the data cannot be directly linked to intervention decisions.
- At present, there is no fluorescence-based device that can be used for proximal and root surface caries.
- They cannot differentiate between active and inactive (arrested) lesions.
- The presence of dental plaque obscures lesion detection.

Application of Bacteria Fluorescence Systems in Caries Management

Some oral microorganisms have the ability to produce porphyrin-like metabolic products that emit red or orange fluorescence when the red extrinsic fluorophores in these bacterial metabolites are excited with the blue (λ = 405 nm) light from the fluorescence-based systems.[4,5] This red fluorescence can be observed in matured dental plaque, calculus, and in more advanced caries lesions (dentinal lesions) and progressive white spots owing to porous surface structures where large molecules can penetrate.[30–33] Some fluorescence-based devices claim to use this principle of red fluorescence to detect and monitor caries activities as a function of bacterial activity (**Figs. 3** and **4**).[13,28,29] Lennon and colleagues[4] demonstrated that, although red fluorescence may detect bacteria that could cause dentin caries, it is not a suitable indicator of the presence and activity of the streptococci involved in initial caries. Furthermore, some of these fluorescence-based devices are recommended by their manufacturers to aid caries excavation during cavity preparation for tooth restoration (see **Fig. 4**).[28,29] This recommendation is based on the claim that observed red fluorescence in carious tissue is an indication of bacteria-infected tissue that needs to be excavated.[32,33] However, bacteria-free demineralized dentin tissue, amenable to recalcification (remineralization) by a cavity liner to protect the pulp, imbibe the porphyrin-like metabolic products from bacteria and as such emits red fluorescence in the absence of bacteria. At the time of writing, there are no independent longitudinal studies supporting these types of claim. More recently, a device was developed, based on this principle of red fluorescence, for the visualization and quantification of bacterial (dental) plaque on tooth surfaces using a Simple Hygiene Score (developed by Inspektor Research Systems, Amsterdam, the Netherlands) that is automatically calculated from fluorescent images (**Fig. 5**).[13] Information about specific fluorescent-based devices is available.[1–5,10–17,20,23–29]

Application of Fluorescence Systems in Oral Surgery

Fluorescence-guided surgery is currently being used in bone resection for patients with chronic osteomyelitis, ORN and MRONJ.[6,7,18,19,34,35] ORN of the jaw is diagnosed as an area of exposed necrotic jaw bone that has failed to heal over a period of 3 to 6 months in an area previously irradiated.[36,37] Although MRONJ is diagnosed as an area of exposed necrotic bone or probe bone either extraorally or intraorally through a fistula of greater than 8 weeks' duration in a patient with a history of antiresorptive or antiangiogenic medication use.[38] ORN and MRONJ are well-known complications in

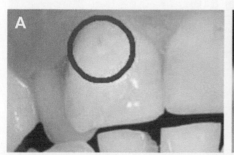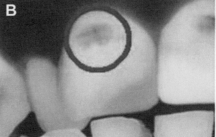

Fig. 3. White light image of an incisor in-vivo with a buccal white spot lesion within the red circle (*A*) and its fluorescent image (*B*) when visualized by one of the commercially available fluorescent-based devices.. (*Courtesy of* Inspektor Research Systems BV, Bussum, Netherlands.)

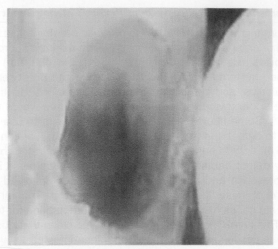

Fig. 4. Red fluorescence being used as a guide for caries excavation during cavity preparation. (*Adapted from* Terrer E, Raskin A, Koubi S, et al. A new concept in restorative dentistry: LIFEDT - light-induced fluorescence evaluator for diagnosis and treatment: part 2 – treatment of dentinal caries. J Contemp Dent Practice 2010;11(1):1–12; with permission.)

patients with cancer who received radiation therapy to the jaws and who are on intravenous bisphosphonates to prevent skeletal-related events, respectively.[37,38] Management of these complications could be very challenging and remains controversial, with no established treatment guidelines in oral surgery and oral medicine. Diverse therapeutic approaches such as conservative use of chlorhexidine gluconate 0.12% or 2.00% rinse with antibiotic therapy (amoxicillin, amoxicillin with clavulanic acid, clindamycin, and/or metronidazole), pentoxifylline and tocopherol, low-level laser therapy, hyperbaric oxygen, and surgery have been used in the management of these complications, with variable clinical outcomes.[37,39]

Clinicians who support the use of surgery for the management of ORN/MRONJ have an argument, based on the fact that infected exposed necrotic bone will not be revitalized. A challenge in the surgical management of ORN/MRONJ is determining to what extent the bone tissue needs to be removed. An incomplete resection risks

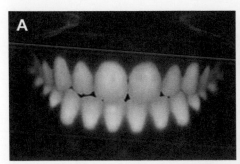
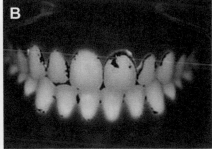

Fig. 5. Red fluorescence being used for visualization and quantitative analysis of dental plaque. (*A*) Original quantitative light-induced fluorescence Red Fluorescence image. (*B*) Visual indication on the original image of all pixels that contributed to the resulting Simple Hygiene Score. (*Courtesy of* Inspektor Research Systems BV, Bussum, Netherlands.)

the possibility of disease progression, whereas an excessive resection risks an unnecessary removal of healthy bone tissue. However, it has long been reported that tetracycline or its derivative "doxycycline" becomes incorporated in healthy vital bone but not in necrotic nonvital bone and can be visualized with appropriate fluorescent light filters.[6,34] When viewed with fluorescent light, healthy vital bone shows a greenish fluorescence and necrotic nonvital bone shows no or significantly lower fluorescence.[18] Based on this principle, some devices have been developed with fluorescent light filters to aid surgeon in applying bone-preserving operative principles during surgical management of patients with ORN/MRONJ. This surgical technique entails patients taking tetracycline or doxycycline over a period of days preoperatively. Intraoperatively, an appropriate fluorescence-based device operating with fluorescent light filter is used to visualize and document bone fluorescence, and areas without fluorescence are resected until natural fluorescence of bone is seen (**Fig. 6**).[6,7,18,19,35] Clinical outcomes with this surgical technique seem to be promising. A recent prospective cohort study reported 86.2% of MRONJ lesions had complete mucosal coverage after first surgery using fluorescence guidance at last follow-up.[35] Information about specific fluorescent-based devices for oral surgery is available.[18,19,34,35]

Application of Fluorescence Systems in Oral Medicine and Oral Pathology

The use of fluorescence in oral medicine and clinical practice has gained much appreciation with the advent of autofluorescence devices marketed for evaluation of the oral mucosa for identification of premalignant and malignant lesions. These devices work by emitting blue light (400–460 nm) onto the oral mucosa and, when viewed through a filter, normal healthy tissue fluoresce a bright green light, whereas suspicious, premalignant and malignant tissue appears dark owing to visual fluorescence loss (**Fig. 7**).

Oral cancer remains a burden to the world at large, making the ninth most common cancer in men in the United States.[40] Squamous cell carcinoma accounts for more than 80% of malignancy in the oral cavity (oral cavity proper and oropharynx).[40] This malignancy is usually preceded by premalignant lesions such as leukoplakia and erythroplakia, exhibiting varying degrees of intraepithelial dysplasia. Survival of this malignancy is greatly dependent on early detection and prevention, although, unfortunately, 70% of new cases of oral squamous cell carcinoma are diagnosed at a late stage.[40]

Autofluorescence devices have been shown to help differentiate normal healthy tissue from premalignant and malignant lesions in the oral cavity, and in identifying the appropriate margin for tumor resection.[2,41,42] However, it has been shown that these devices cannot differentiate other benign mucosal lesions from premalignant and malignant lesions. Benign mucosal lesions such as inflammatory conditions, traumatic ulcerations, lymphoid-rich areas, and melanin pigments would appear dark (visual fluorescence loss) on autofluorescence (**Fig. 8**), giving rise to a lot of false-positive readings warranting unneeded biopsies on patients. Conventional visual oral examination was demonstrated to be more accurate in discriminating benign mucosal lesions from premalignant lesions in a study that evaluated 130 patients comparing conventional visual oral examination and the examination using one of the fluorescence-based devices with histopathologic evaluation as the gold standard.[9] In this study, all mucosal abnormalities detected by the fluorescence-based device were detected by conventional visual oral examination.[9] However, the fluorescence-based device showed false-positive and false-negative readings as previously reported in other studies.[9,43] Thus, a recent evidence-based clinical practice guideline from the American Dental Association does not recommend the use of autofluorescence devices as diagnostic adjuncts in the evaluation of oral premalignant lesions in adults with clinically evident, seemingly innocuous, or suspicious lesions (fourth recommendation).[21]

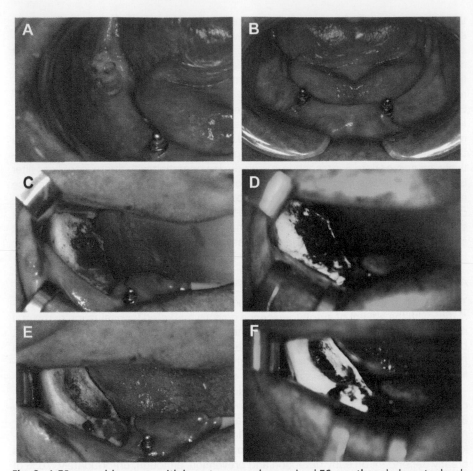

Fig. 6. A 58-year-old woman with breast cancer who received 56 months zoledronate developed a medication-related osteonecrosis of the jaw in her left mandible (region 37/38 mainly lingual aspect). The illustration depicts the clinical intraoral situation before (*A*) and 3 months after surgery (*B*). The intraoperative clinical and fluorescence view before removal of the necrotic bone (*C, D*) and after the removal of necrotic bone and smoothening of sharp bony edges (*E, F*) are also illustrated. Note the weak green fluorescence in the lingual aspect region 37/38 corresponding with the necrotic bone area (*D*) as well as the reddish fluorescence in this area corresponding to the bacterial infection of this region before removal of the necrotic and infected bone parts as well as the homogenous greenish fluorescence after the removal and the absence of red fluorescence after the removal of necrotic bone parts. (*From* Otto S, Ristow O, Pache C, et al. Fluorescence-guided surgery for the treatment of medication-related osteonecrosis of the jaw: a prospective cohort study. J Craniomaxillofac Surg 2016;44(8):1076; with permission.)

Information about specific fluorescent-based devices for oral surgery is available elsewhere.

NEAR-INFRARED LIGHT TRANSILLUMINATION CAMERA SYSTEMS

Based on the discovery that enamel is highly transparent in the NIR,[44] the high potential of the NIR for imaging caries lesions on both proximal and occlusal surfaces was

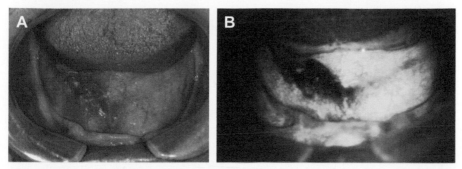

Fig. 7. (*A*) Conventional visual oral examination showing a tumor at the floor of the mouth, and (*B*) VELscope image showing visual fluorescence loss in the green light spectrum in the tumor area. (*From* Burian E, Schulz C, Probst F, et al. Fluorescence based characterization of early oral squamous cell carcinoma using the Visually Enhanced Light Scope technique. J Craniomaxillofac Surg 2017;45(9):1528; with permission.)

demonstrated.[45] Also demonstrated was that novel imaging configurations such as occlusal transillumination imaging can be used to image lesions on both occlusal and proximal surfaces.[45] A plot of the attenuation of light in enamel and water is shown in **Fig. 9** as a function of wavelength from 400 to 2000 nm.[44,46] Light scattering increases by 2 to 3 orders of magnitude with demineralization at a Δ of 1300 nm, indicating that high contrast in transillumination between sound and carious tissues is found near a Δ of 1300 nm as well.[47]

The first NIR proximal transillumination images of natural lesions were acquired at 1310 nm.[48] Subsequent measurements were performed at shorter wavelengths where conventional low cost silicon based detectors can be used. The contrast of simulated lesions in sections of enamel from 2- to 7-mm thickness was compared for visible, 830-nm, and 1310-nm wavelengths.[49] The image contrast for these wavelengths is plotted in **Fig. 10**. The contrast was higher at 830 nm than the visible, but the contrast

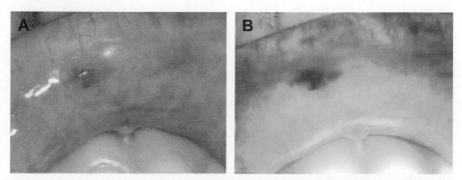

Fig. 8. Conventional visual oral examination showing erythema and ulceration of the upper labial mucosa (*A*), and same lesion demonstrating visual fluorescence loss on examination with VELscope (*B*). This clinical finding was consistent with a traumatic etiology and lesion resolved on follow-up. (*Adapted from* McNamara KK, Martin BD, Evans EW, et al. The role of direct visual fluorescent examination (VELscope) in routine screening for potentially malignant oral mucosal lesions. Oral Surg Oral Med Oral Pathol Oral Radiol 2012;114(5):640; with permission.)

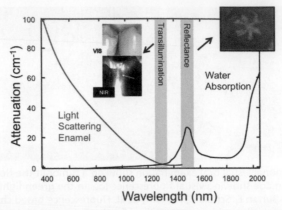

Fig. 9. The attenuation coefficient for dental enamel (*red*) and the absorption coefficient of water (*blue*) in the visible and near-infrared. An established proximal caries lesion (*yellow arrow*) revealed by transillumination. Best wavelengths for transillumination (1300 nm) and best wavelengths for reflectance (1450 and 1940 nm) and example images are shown for each modality. (*Data from* Refs.[44,46,62])

was highest at 1310-nm and only at 1310 nm were the lesions visible through 6 to 7 mm of enamel.[49]

After these studies, multiple commercial NIR clinical imaging devices have been introduced; CariVu (Dexis, Hatfield, PA) which uses NIR occlusal transillumination with 780-nm light[50] and the Vistacam IX (PROXI) from Durr Dental (Bietigheim-Bissingen, Germany), which uses NIR reflectance at 850 nm.

NIR light transillumination camera systems are based on the principle that light intensity can be reduced by absorption (eg, photons are lost to the hard tissue or the caries lesion) or scattering, in which the direction of the photons is changed without

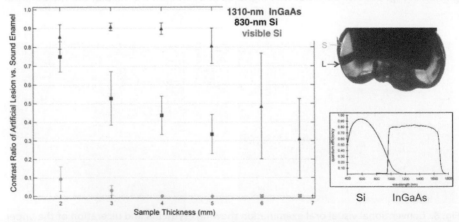

Fig. 10. Plot of the mean ± standard deviation lesion contrast $(I_S-I_L)/I_S$ versus sample thickness for simulated lesions calculated for samples of varying thickness (n = 3 samples per thickness). Example of sample shown in inset. The spectral responsivity of Si and InGaAs detectors is also shown. L, lesion; S, sound. (*Adapted from* Jones G, Jones RS, Fried D, editors. Transillumination of interproximal caries lesions with 830-nm light. Lasers in Dentistry X. San Jose: SPIE; 2004; vol. 5313. p. 17–22; with permission.)

loss of energy. In the NIR range of light (700–1500 nm), wavelengths are significantly longer than in the range of visible light, and longer wavelengths scatter less, and thus can penetrate deeper into the tooth tissue.[47] With NIR light transillumination, each tooth tissue (enamel or dentin) will be uniformly illuminated, with enamel appearing to be transparent while dentin scatters light more strongly; thus, the 2 tissues can be distinguished.[45,51] When tooth tissue is demineralized at the earliest stage of caries, this results in a higher scattering coefficient,[47] thus reducing light intensity, and as such the presence of caries shows as a dark area at the marginal ridge for proximal caries (**Fig. 11**) or at occlusal surface for occlusal caries (**Fig. 12**). NIR wavelengths longer than 1300 nm may enable improved performance for the transillumination of occlusal caries lesions whereas 1300 nm seems to be best for the transillumination of proximal surfaces.[52] The contrast between sound and demineralized enamel is greatest in the NIR owing to the minimal scattering of sound enamel and this is exploited for reflectance imaging of early demineralization.[45] The first NIR reflectance study was carried out by Wu and Fried,[51] and they found that the contrast of early demineralization was significantly higher at 1310-nm than in the visible range. Zakian and colleagues[53] acquired hyperspectral reflectance images of occlusal caries lesions and demonstrated that multiwavelength images could be used to aid diagnosis. The greatest contrast is achieved at longer NIR wavelengths coincident with greater water absorption.[54] Water in the underlying dentin and surrounding sound enamel absorbs the deeply penetrating light and reduces the reflectivity in sound areas and this in turn results in higher contrast between sound and demineralized enamel. The highest contrast is at 1450 nm, where there is a water absorption band (see **Fig. 9**). The greater contrast at 1450 nm can be seen in **Fig. 13**, which shows a reflection images at various wavelengths in addition to quantitative light-induced fluorescence.[54] Stains are not visible in NIR images of occlusal surfaces because the organic molecules responsible for pigmentation absorb poorly in the NIR, making it easier to identify areas of demineralization,[55] and thus improving specificity with NIR-based devices. With NIR in the 1460-nm range, composite restoration is much lighter than the surrounding enamel, so there is potential for imaging around composite restorations for presence of caries around restorations (secondary caries).[52,56]

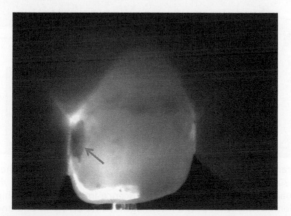

Fig. 11. An established proximal caries lesion (*arrow*) revealed by a near-infrared light transillumination device. (*Adapted from* Söchtig F, Hickel R, Kühnisch J. Caries detection and diagnostics with near-infrared light transillumination: clinical experiences. Quintessence Int 2014;45(6):531–8; with permission.)

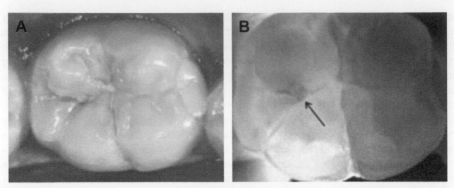

Fig. 12. (*A*) A clinically sound occlusal tooth surface with hidden occlusal caries lesion revealed by a near-infrared light transillumination device as a (*B*) circumscribed area of significant changed occlusal translucence (*arrow*). (*Adapted from* Söchtig F, Hickel R, Kühnisch J. Caries detection and diagnostics with near-infrared light transillumination: clinical experiences. Quintessence Int 2014;45(6):531–8; with permission.)

In the first NIR clinical study in 2009, it was demonstrated that approximal lesions that appeared on radiographs could be detected with NIR proximal and occlusal transillumination with similar sensitivity.[55] **Fig. 14** shows radiographs and proximal and occlusal transillumination images acquired at 1310 nm from that study. Even though the sensitivity of radiographs is not very high,[45,56] most studies indicate

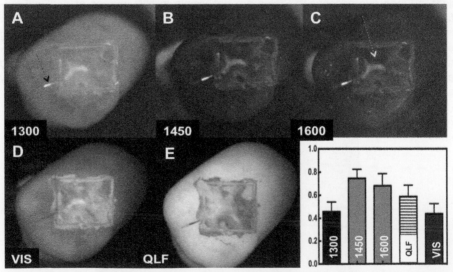

Fig. 13. Near-infrared (NIR) reflectance images of demineralization on the occlusal surface of a tooth, (*A*) 1300 nm, (*B*) 1460 nm, and (*C*) 1600 nm, along with (*D*) visible reflectance image and (*E*) quantitative light-induced fluorescence image. Note the high contrast area of more severe demineralization in the NIR images (*white arrow* in *C*) along with the residual natural demineralization and stain outside the 4 × 4-mm window (*black arrow* in *A*). (*Adapted from* Fried WA, Chan KH, Fried D, et al. High contrast reflectance imaging of simulated lesions on tooth occlusal surfaces at near-IR wavelengths. Lasers Surg Med 2013;45:533–41; with permission.)

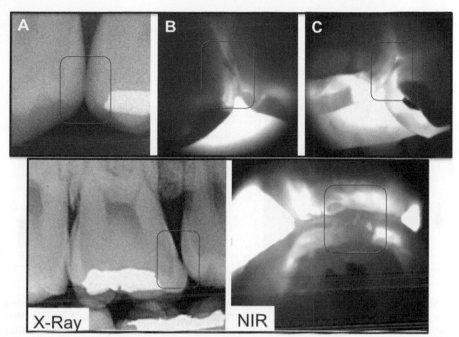

Fig. 14. (*Top*) Radiographs (*A*) and in vivo proximal transillumination images at 1300-nm, buccal (*B*) and lingual (*C*) views of the contact point. (*Bottom*) Radiographic and in vivo occlusal transillumination image (near-infrared [NIR]) at 1300 nm of a tooth from the first NIR clinical study. (*Adapted from* Staninec M, Lee C, Darling CL, et al. In vivo near-IR imaging of approximal dental decay at 1310 nm. Lasers Surg Med 2010;42(4):292–8; with permission.)

that the specificity of radiographs is greater than 90%, which made it a suitable standard for comparison for the first test of this new imaging technology. The first clinical studies using a commercial device operating at shorter wavelengths (780 nm) shows promise for detecting proximal caries.[50,57] The NIR is also well-suited for the detection of cracks and fractures.[58] In a recent clinical study using both NIR reflectance and transillumination,[59] images of premolar teeth were taken before extraction at wavelengths from 1500 to 1700 nm. The diagnostic performance of the NIR exceeded radiography for lesions on both proximal and occlusal surfaces.

NIR reflectance imaging can also be used with dehydration in a similar fashion to quantitative light-induced fluorescence to assess changes in lesion activity and severity. At wavelengths longer than 1400 nm, where water absorption is high, there are very large changes in contrast with dehydration and the magnitude of that change varies with the degree of remineralization.[60] This finding is demonstrated in **Fig. 15**: NIR reflectance at 1450 nm was able to detect changes in remineralization.[60]

Recent clinical studies showed the application of NIR light transillumination has the potential to reduce the use of bitewing radiography for detecting proximal and occlusal caries,[50,57] in addition to its ability to detect cracks and fractures. Thus, NIR light imaging methods have great potential as an aid for clinical caries detection and assessment, considering the following benefits currently associated with these systems.

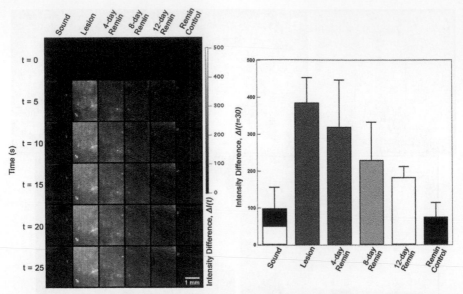

Fig. 15. The intensity change (ΔI) in reflectance at 1450 nm in bovine enamel during forced air-drying after demineralization and remineralization. (*Left*) Images of the 6 sample windows after different drying times. Note the greatest degree of change occurs in the first 5 s between t = 0 and t = 5. (*Right*) Marked differences in ΔI were observed after remineralization. Bars of same color are statistically similar (P>.05; n = 30). (*Adapted from* Lee RC, Darling CL, Fried D. Assessment of remineralization via measurement of dehydration rates with thermal and near-IR reflectance imaging. J Dent 2015;43:1032–42; with permission.)

- They are highly sensitive, thus enabling them to detect caries lesion at its earliest stage of development.
- At wavelengths beyond 1200 nm, NIR images are free of interference from stain and the lesion contrast increases with lesion depth in transillumination images.[61] Therefore, the NIR has great potential for improving the diagnosis of questionable occlusal lesions, those that do not appear on radiographs.[61]
- These systems may be able to indicate the depth of proximal caries but not that of occlusal lesions; thus, they proved to be the best adjunct to bitewing radiographs.[57]
- These systems are useful for detecting hidden proximal and occlusal caries, fractures, and cracks
- Most NIR light transillumination devices are able to show digital images of the tooth surface and the associated lesions, thus facilitating patient education and motivation with digitized images of the caries lesion (see **Figs. 11** and **12**).

With innovative improvement to overcome the following currently associated drawbacks, NIR light transillumination systems have the potential to be the best replacement for radiograph as a diagnostic tool for dental caries management.

- They cannot detect caries underneath restorations owing to the limitation in the penetration of light at the current wavelength used in the existing devices.
- Stains interfere at wavelengths below 1200 nm to produce false positives and prevent accurate measurement of lesion severity. Stains may completely mask demineralization in the pits and fissures at these shorter wavelengths.[61]

- They cannot differentiate between active and arrested lesions
- Because NIR imaging is a new technology and it is more sensitive than radiographs, it should be approached with care to avoid false positives and overtreatment.

REFERENCES

1. Heinrich-Weltzien R, Kühnisch J, van der Veen MH, et al. Quantitative light-induced fluorescence (QLF™) - a potential method for the dental practitioner. Quintessence Int 2003;34:181–8.
2. ten Bosch JJ. Light scattering and related methods in caries diagnosis. In: Stookey GK, editor. Early detection of dental caries: Proceedings of the 1st Annual Indiana Conference. Indianapolis (IN): Indiana University Press; 1996. p. 81–90.
3. de Josselin de Jong E, Hall AF, van der Veen MH. Quantitative light-induced fluorescence detection method. A Monte Carlo simulation model. In: Stookey GK, editor. Early detection of dental caries: Proceedings of the 1st Annual Indiana Conference. Indianapolis (IN): Indiana University Press; 1996. p. 91–104.
4. Lennon AM, Buchalla W, Brune L, et al. The ability of selected oral microorganisms to emit red fluorescence. Caries Res 2006;40:2–5.
5. Könlg K, Flemming G, Hibst R. Laser-induced autofluorescence spectroscopy of dental caries. Cell Mol Biol (Noisy-le-grand) 1998;44:1293–300.
6. Harvey BR, Ephros H, Defalco RJ. Tetracycline bone labeling in surgical management of chronic osteomyelitis: a case report. J Oral Maxillofac Surg 2004;62: 752–4.
7. Pautke C, Tischer T, Neff A, et al. In vivo tetracycline labeling of bone: an intraoperative aid in the surgical therapy of osteoradionecrosis of the mandible. Oral Surg Oral Med Oral Pathol Oral Radiol Endod 2006;102:e10–3.
8. Burian E, Schulz C, Probst F, et al. Fluorescence based characterization of early oral squamous cell carcinoma using the Visually Enhanced Light Scope technique. J Craniomaxillofac Surg 2017;45:1526–30.
9. McNamara KK, Martin BD, Evans EW, et al. The role of direct visual fluorescent examination (VELscope) in routine screening for potentially malignant oral mucosal lesions. Oral Surg Oral Med Oral Pathol Oral Radiol 2012;114:636–43.
10. Amaechi BT, Higham SM. Quantitative light-induced fluorescence: a potential tool for general dental assessment. J Biomed Opt 2002;7:7–13.
11. van der Veen MH, de Josselin de Jong E. Application of quantitative light-induced fluorescence for assessing early caries lesions. Monogr Oral Sci 2000; 17:144–62.
12. Pretty IA. Caries detection and diagnosis: novel technologies. J Dent 2006;34: 727–39.
13. de Josselin de Jong E. Quantitative light-induced fluorescence: theoretical background. Available at: http://www.inspektor.nl/index.php/evidence/background/. Accessed October 20, 2010.
14. Han SY, Kim BR, Ko HY, et al. Assessing the use of quantitative light-induced fluorescence-digital as a clinical plaque assessment. Photodiagnosis Photodyn Ther 2016;13:34–9.
15. van der Veen MH, Volgenant CM, Keijser B, et al. Dynamics of red fluorescent dental plaque during experimental gingivitis—a cohort study. J Dent 2016;48: 71–6.

16. Han SY, Kim BR, Ko HY, et al. Validity and reliability of autofluorescence-based quantification method of dental plaque. Photodiagnosis Photodyn Ther 2015; 12:587–91.

17. Ku HM, Jun MK, Kim JH, et al. Explaining the red fluorescence evident on the surface of failed dental implants: case reports. Implant Dent 2016;25:1–5.

18. Pautke C, Bauer F, Tischer T, et al. Fluorescence-guided bone resection in bisphosphonate-associated osteonecrosis of the jaws. J Oral Maxillofac Surg 2009;67:471–6.

19. Pautke C, Bauer F, Otto S, et al. Fluorescence-guided bone resection in bisphosphonate-related osteonecrosis of the jaws: first clinical results of a prospective pilot study. J Oral Maxillofac Surg 2011;69:84–91.

20. Amaechi BT. Emerging technologies for diagnosis of dental caries: the road so far. J Appl Phys 2009;105:1–9.

21. Lingen MW, Abt E, Agrawal N, et al. Evidence-based clinical practice guideline for the evaluation of potentially malignant disorders in the oral cavity: a report of the American Dental Association. J Am Dent Assoc 2017;148:712–727 e10.

22. Amaechi BT. Using technology to aid in early detection and diagnosis of caries lesions. MetLife® quality resource guide. 2nd edition. Bridgewater (NJ): MetLife Dental; 2016. p. 13. Booklet.

23. van der Veen MH, de Josselin de Jong E. The introduction of a new parameter Q for incipient caries measurement with QLF. Caries Res 1999;33:318–20.

24. van der Veen MH, de Josselin de Jong E. Technical manual for quantitative light-induced fluorescence, version 2000, Inspektor Research Systems BV, Amsterdam, The Netherlands. 2005.

25. Ferreira Zandoná AG, Isaacs RL, van der Veen MH, et al. Indiana pilot clinical study of quantitative light fluorescence. In: Stookey GK, editor. Early detection of dental caries II: Proceedings of the 4th Annual Indiana Conference. Indianapolis (IN): Indiana University Press; 2000. p. 219–30.

26. Stookey GK, Isaacs RL, Minami M, et al. Clinical assessment of remineralization from fluoride varnish treatments. J Dent Res 2009;88(Sp. Iss A) [abstract: 1167].

27. Stookey GK, Isaacs RL, White VA, et al. Clinical monitoring of white spot lesions in children: 12-Month Results. J Dent Res 2011;90(Sp. Iss A) [abstract: 3371].

28. Terrer E, Raskin A, Koubi S, et al. New concept in restorative dentistry: LIFEDT-light- induced fluorescence evaluator for diagnosis and treatment: part 1 – Diagnosis and treatment of initial occlusal caries. J Contemp Dent Pract 2009;10: 1–12.

29. Terrer E, Raskin A, Koubi S, et al. A new concept in restorative dentistry: LIFEDT-light- induced fluorescence evaluator for diagnosis and treatment: part 2 – Treatment of dentinal caries. J Contemp Dent Pract 2010;11:1–12.

30. Buchalla W. Comparative fluorescence spectroscopy shows differences in non-cavitated enamel lesions. Caries Res 2005;39:150–6.

31. Buchalla W, Lennon AM, Attin T. Comparative fluorescence spectroscopy of root caries lesions. Eur J Oral Sci 2004;112:490–6.

32. Lennon AM, Buchalla W, Switalski L, et al. Residual caries detection using visible fluorescence. Caries Res 2002;36:315–9.

33. Lennon AM, Attin T, Martens S, et al. Fluorescence-aided caries excavation (FACE), caries detector, and conventional caries excavation in primary teeth. Pediatr Dent 2009;31:316–9.

34. Otto S, Baumann S, Ehrenfeld M, et al. Successful surgical management of osteonecrosis of the jaw due to RANK-ligand inhibitor treatment using fluorescence guided bone resection. J Craniomaxillofac Surg 2013;41:694–8.

35. Otto S, Ristow O, Pache C, et al. Fluorescence-guided surgery for the treatment of medication-related osteonecrosis of the jaw: a prospective cohort study. J Craniomaxillofac Surg 2016;44:1073–80.

36. Marx RE. Osteoradionecrosis: a new concept of its pathophysiology. J Oral Maxillofac Surg 1983;41:283–8.

37. Owosho AA, Tsai CJ, Lee RS, et al. The prevalence and risk factors associated with osteoradionecrosis of the jaw in oral and oropharyngeal cancer patients treated with intensity-modulated radiation therapy (IMRT): the Memorial Sloan Kettering Cancer Center experience. Oral Oncol 2017;64:44–51.

38. Ruggiero SL, Dodson TB, Fantasia J, et al. American Association of Oral and Maxillofacial Surgeons position paper on medication-related osteonecrosis of the jaw–2014 update. J Oral Maxillofac Surg 2014;72:1938–56.

39. Watters AL, Hansen HJ, Williams T, et al. Intravenous bisphosphonate-related osteonecrosis of the jaw: long-term follow-up of 109 patients. Oral Surg Oral Med Oral Pathol Oral Radiol 2013;115:192–200.

40. Siegel RL, Miller KD, Jemal A. Cancer statistics, 2017. CA Cancer J Clin 2017;67:7–30.

41. Lane PM, Gilhuly T, Whitehead P, et al. Simple device for the direct visualization of oral-cavity tissue fluorescence. J Biomed Opt 2006;11:024006.

42. Poh CF, Ng SP, Williams PM, et al. Direct fluorescence visualization of clinically occult high- risk oral premalignant disease using a simple hand-held device. Head Neck 2007;29:71–6.

43. Mehrotra R, Singh M, Thomas S, et al. A cross-sectional study evaluating chemiluminescence and autofluorescence in the detection of clinically innocuous precancerous and cancerous oral lesions. J Am Dent Assoc 2010;141(2):151–6.

44. Fried D, Glena RE, Featherstone JD, et al. Nature of light scattering in dental enamel and dentin at visible and near-infrared wavelengths. Appl Opt 1995;34(7):1278–85.

45. Staninec M, Lee C, Darling CL, et al. In vivo near-IR imaging of approximal dental decay at 1310 nm. Lasers Surg Med 2010;42(4):292–8.

46. Hale GM, Querry MR. Optical constants of water in the 200-nm to 200-μm wavelength region. Appl Opt 1973;12:555–63.

47. Darling CL, Huynh GD, Fried D. Light scattering properties of natural and artificially demineralized dental enamel at 1310-nm. J Biomed Opt 2006;11(3):34023.

48. Jones RS, Huynh GD, Jones GC, et al. Near-IR transillumination at 1310-nm for the imaging of early dental caries. Opt Express 2003;11(18):2259–65.

49. Jones G, Jones RS, Fried D, editors. Transillumination of interproximal caries lesions with 830-nm light. Lasers in dentistry X, vol. 5313. San Jose (CA): SPIE; 2004. p. 17–22.

50. Kühnisch J, Söchtig F, Pitchika V, et al. In vivo validation of near-infrared light transillumination for interproximal dentin caries detection. Clin Oral Investig 2016;20(4):821–9.

51. Wu J, Fried D. High contrast near-infrared polarized reflectance images of demineralization on tooth buccal and occlusal surfaces at lambda = 1310 nm. Lasers Surg Med 2009;41:208–13.

52. Chung S, Fried D, Staninec M, et al. Multispectral near-IR reflectance and transillumination imaging of teeth. Biomed Opt Express 2011;2(10):2804–14.

53. Zakian C, Pretty I, Ellwood R. Near-infrared hyperspectral imaging of teeth for dental caries detection. J Biomed Opt 2009;14(6):064047.

54. Fried WA, Chan KH, Fried D, et al. High contrast reflectance imaging of simulated lesions on tooth occlusal surfaces at near-IR wavelengths. Lasers Surg Med 2013;45:533–41.
55. Bühler CM, Ngaotheppitak P, Fried D. Imaging of occlusal dental caries (decay) with near-IR light at 1310-nm. Opt Express 2005;13(2):573–82.
56. Simon JC, AL S, Lee RC, et al. Near-infrared imaging of secondary caries lesions around composite restorations at wavelengths from 1300-1700-nm. Dent Mater 2016;32(4):587–95.
57. Söchtig F, Hickel R, Kühnisch J. Caries detection and diagnostics with near-infrared light transillumination: clinical experiences. Quintessence Int 2014; 45(6):531–8.
58. Fried WA, Simon JC, Lucas S, et al. editors. Near-IR imaging of cracks in teeth. Lasers in Dentistry XX; 2014: Proceedings of SPIE 89290(Q):1–6.
59. Simon JC, Lucas SA, Lee RC, et al. Near-IR transillumination and reflectance imaging at 1300-nm and 1500-1700-nm for in vivo caries detection. Lasers Surg Med 2016;48(6):828–36.
60. Lee RC, Darling CL, Fried D. Assessment of remineralization via measurement of dehydration rates with thermal and near-IR reflectance imaging. J Dent 2015;43: 1032–42.
61. Simon JC, Kang H, Staninec M, et al. Near-IR and CP-OCT imaging of suspected occlusal caries lesions. Lasers Surg Med 2017;49(3):215–24.
62. Jones RS, Fried D. Attenuation of 1310-nm and 1550-nm laser light through sound dental enamel. In: Lasers in Dentistry VIII; 2002. Proc SPIE. vol. 4610. p. 187–90.

Multidetector Row Computed Tomography in Maxillofacial Imaging

Anita Gohel, BDS, PhD[a],*, Masafumi Oda, DDS, PhD[b,c],
Amol S. Katkar, MD[d], Osamu Sakai, MD, PhD[b,e,f]

KEYWORDS

- Multidetector row CT • Maxillofacial • Imaging • Dual-energy CT • Perfusion CT
- Texture analysis

KEY POINTS

- Multidetector row CT (MDCT) is useful for the diagnosis of odontogenic and nonodontogenic cysts and tumors, fibro-osseous lesions, inflammation, malignancy, metastatic lesions, developmental abnormalities, and maxillofacial trauma.
- Perfusion MDCT aids in lesion characterization, staging, and tumor prognosis based on vascularity and also helps in monitoring the response of various treatment regimens.
- Dual-energy CT imaging allows for material differentiation and characterization by creating monochromatic energy images and can minimize metal artifacts.
- CT texture analysis is a postprocessing technique that can provide a quantitative means of extracting image features that are useful for comparative analyses.

CT has proved an invaluable diagnostic imaging modality for many maxillofacial clinical applications. Since its introduction in 1972, several improvements have occurred as decreased acquisition time and enhanced image quality.[1,2] Shorter acquisition time reduces motion artifacts caused by breathing, swallowing and patient movements. In the mid-1990s, the introduction of multidetector row CT (MDCT) led to submillimeter spatial

Disclosure Statement: None (A. Gohel, M. Oda and A.S. Katkar); Consultant, Boston Imaging Core Lab, LLC (unrelated to this article) (O. Sakai).
[a] Oral and Maxillofacial Pathology and Radiology, College of Dentistry, The Ohio State University, 3165 Postle Hall, 305 West 12th Avenue, Columbus, OH 43210-1267, USA; [b] Department of Radiology, Boston Medical Center, Boston University School of Medicine, 820 Harrison Avenue, Boston, MA 02118, USA; [c] Division of Oral and Maxillofacial Radiology, Kyushu Dental University, 2-6-1 Manazuru, Kokurakita-ku, Kitakyushu 803-8580, Japan; [d] Department of Radiology, Brook Army Medical Center, 3851 Roger Brooke Drive, Fort Sam Houston, TX 78234-6200, USA; [e] Department of Radiation Oncology, Boston Medical Center, Boston University School of Medicine, 820 Harrison Avenue, Boston, MA 02118, USA; [f] Department of Otolaryngology–Head and Neck Surgery, Boston Medical Center, Boston University School of Medicine, 820 Harrison Avenue, Boston, MA 02118, USA
* Corresponding author.
E-mail address: gohel.6@osu.edu

Dent Clin N Am 62 (2018) 453–465
https://doi.org/10.1016/j.cden.2018.03.005
0011-8532/18/© 2018 Elsevier Inc. All rights reserved.

dental.theclinics.com

resolution scans. MDCT has transformed CT from transaxial cross-sectional imaging into a truly 3-D imaging. The images are obtained at a high resolution and thinner sections as volume data, leading to multiplanar reformation and near isotropic images at a high acquisition rate.[3–5] One of the other major advantages of MDCT over single-detector row CT is the increase in efficiency and flexibility of the use of contrast medium.[4]

Nonenhanced MDCT scan can delineate bony, soft tissue, and air space abnormalities as well as calcifications. Contrast-enhanced scans may be added to demonstrate vascular lesions or abnormal vascular permeability in inflammatory or neoplastic neovascularity.[4] The contrast agent can be used more efficiently in an MDCT scan. Compared with 120 mL of the standard contrast (300 mg iodine/mL), a 90 mL of higher concentration contrast (400 mg iodine/mL) may produce better contrast enhancement in tumors and increase contrast between normal soft tissue and the tumor. The shorter image acquisition time enables image acquisition at a high spatial resolution at multiple and exactly defined phases of contrast enhancement.[4,6]

In the maxillofacial region, MDCT offers superior soft tissue characterization compared with cone-beam CT images and is useful for the diagnosis of odontogenic and nonodontogenic cysts and tumors, fibro-osseous lesions, inflammation, malignancy, metastatic lesions, developmental abnormalities, and maxillofacial trauma.[4,7,8]

MULTIDETECTOR ROW CT IN THE DIAGNOSIS OF BENIGN ODONTOGENIC AND NONODONTOGENIC LESIONS

MDCT scans can demonstrate the extent of the lesions, expansion in all 3 planes and the boundary of these benign lesions. The expansile lesion as well as water-density within a cyst with no extraosseous lesion is noted in a dentigerous cyst (**Fig. 1**). Low-density cystic areas with few isodensity regions representing soft tissue in a CT image is seen in an ameloblastoma (**Fig. 2**). The aggressiveness of the lesion can be appreciated by erosion of the cortical plate or tooth root. Contrast-enhanced CT depicts the enhanced soft tissue within the lesion.[9]

Odontogenic myxoma is also an aggressive multilocular expansile lesion. The straight septa, a distinctive finding, can be seen in CT images (**Fig. 3**). Odontogenic keratocysts are unilocular or multilocular lesions most commonly located in the

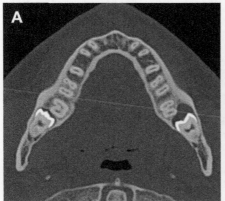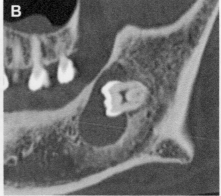

Fig. 1. Dentigerous cyst in a 32-year-old man. Axial (*A*) and sagittal (*B*) CT images show a unilocular lucent lesion associated with the crown of the left mandibular third molar. There is no aggressive expansile change or destruction of the buccal or lingual cortex adjacent to the lesion. Note the sclerosis of surrounding bone indicative of an inflammatory response.

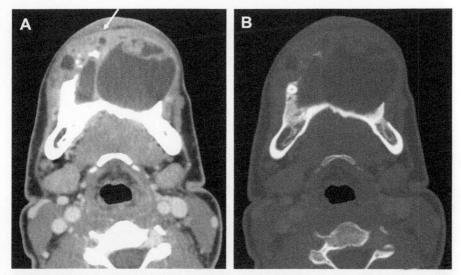

Fig. 2. Ameloblastoma in a 35-year-old man presenting with anterior mandible swelling. Axial soft tissue (*A*) and bone (*B*) reconstructed contrast-enhanced CT images show a multi-septated, lytic, and expansile mostly cystic lesion demonstrating enhancing nodular soft tissue component (*arrow*) peripherally centered in the mandibular symphysis. The lesion erodes through the labial surface of the mandible.

posterior mandible, and are noted to grow with minimal expansion, and significant expansion may occur in the ramus (**Fig. 4**).

The nonenhanced CT reveals phleboliths seen in many low-flow vascular lesions, including venous malformations (**Fig. 5**A). Contrast-enhanced CT can show the enhancement of a vascular lesion (**Fig. 5**B).

MULTIDETECTOR ROW CT IN THE DIAGNOSIS OF AGGRESSIVE LESIONS

Aggressive lesions usually have irregular margin and may be permeative lesions with invasive or infiltrative borders and a wide zone of transition. The presence of a soft tissue component in these images with a bone lesion also is suggestive of a malignant

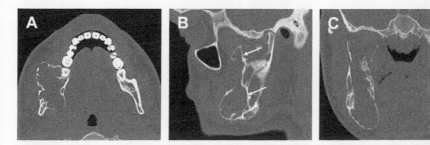

Fig. 3. Odontogenic myxoma in a 24-year-old man presenting with right cheek swelling. Axial (*A*), sagittal (*B*), and coronal (*C*) CT images show a large expansile lesion in the right mandibular angle to ramus. The significant expansion and erosion of cortical bone reflects aggressiveness of the lesion. Note the straight septa (*arrows*), a distinctive finding of odontogenic myxoma.

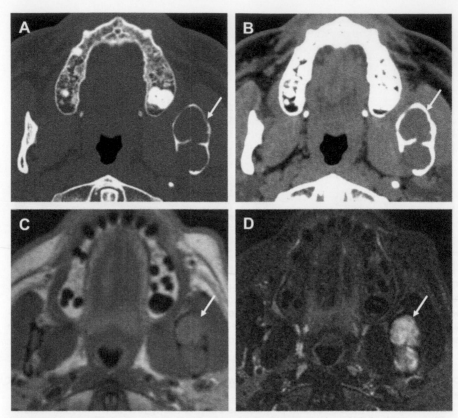

Fig. 4. Odontogenic keratocyst in a 64-year-old man presented with left cheek swelling. Axial CT (*A*, *B*) shows multicystic and multiloculated expansile lesion involving the left mandibular ramus (*arrows*). Axial T1-weighted MR image (*C*) shows low-to-intermediate signal, and T2-weighted MR image (*D*) shows heterogeneous intermediate-to-high signal within the lesion reflecting keratinized contents (*arrows*).

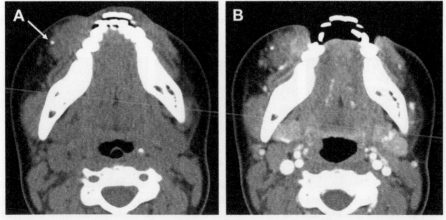

Fig. 5. Venous malformation in a 12-year-old girl. Noncontrast CT (*A*) shows a soft tissue mass in the right buccal space. A nodular calcification, phlebolith (*arrow*), is demonstrated. Contrast-enhanced CT (*B*) shows the lesion heterogeneously and partially enhanced.

process. Periosteal changes, such as bone destruction with no periosteal reactions, laminated peripheral periosteal reaction (Codman triangle), and a spiculated periosteal reaction (sunray pattern) may be appreciated in MDCT scans.[10,11] Although there is considerable overlap, at times the subtype of periosteal reaction can be suggestive of a certain disease. Solid periosteal reaction is a nonaggressive form that is primarily seen with benign, slow processes. The laminated appearance is seen in a variety of lesions, including osteomyelitis and sarcomas. The amorphous, spiculated, or sunburst-like periosteal reaction and Codman triangles are usually seen in malignant lesions.[12] Malignant lesions, such as squamous cell carcinoma, can cause bone disruption and extend into the surrounding space (**Fig. 6**A, B). Contrast-enhanced CT aids in the evaluation of lymph nodes (**Fig. 6**C).

Advances in PET/CT has had a significant impact in the maxillofacial cancer diagnosis. [18]Fluorine-2-fluoro-2-deoxy-D-glucose (^{18}F-FDG) is a short-lived radiopharmaceutical used for PET/CT scanning and is an important diagnostic tool to evaluate head and neck squamous cell carcinomas for assessment of the primary and secondary tumor, cervical lymph nodes, distant metastases, treatment response, and post-therapy follow-up.[13,14] ^{18}F-FDG uptake depends on glucose metabolism and is seen in several normal tissues with wide variability of the normal pattern, including the brain, salivary glands, cervical muscles, and lymphoid tissue as well as in benign tumors, such as Warthin tumor. One of the limitations of this method is the false-positive results due to inflammation, such as inflamed lymph node or periodontitis.[15] Significant increase of FDG uptake can be seen in the primary lesion site and lymph nodes in squamous cell carcinoma (**Fig. 6**D, E).

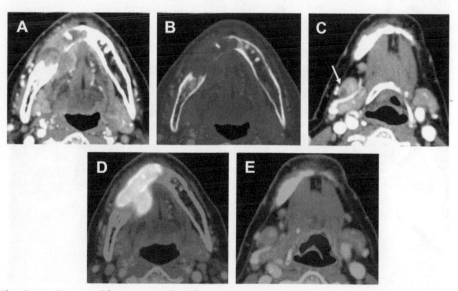

Fig. 6. An 81-year-old woman with right gingival squamous cell carcinoma. Soft tissue (*A*) and bone (*B*) reconstructed contrast-enhanced CT images show a lesion disrupting and replacing the right mandibular body. Medially, there is extension into the sublingual space. Axial image of the lower level (*C*) shows an enlarged, metastatic level IB node with internal necrosis (*arrow*). PET/CT image at the primary lesion level (*D*) shows significant increase of FDG uptake (maximum standardized uptake value 19.5) within the lesion. The image of the lower level (*E*) demonstrates increased FDG uptake (maximum standardized uptake value 5.9) in the right level IB lymph node.

Perineural spread has been reported in squamous cell carcinoma, adenoid cystic carcinoma (**Fig. 7**A), mucoepidermoid carcinoma, desmoplastic melanoma, and non-Hodgkin lymphoma.[16,17] Multiplanar imaging is essential to evaluate nerve canals, fissures, fossae, and foramina (**Fig. 7**B, C). It is often difficult to diagnose perineural spread because 40% of patients may be asymptomatic.[17] The detection of perineural tumor spread is critical for proper treatment planning. Identifying loss of normal fat and thickening of the involved nerve is a keep concept to diagnose perineural tumor spread on CT or MRI (see **Fig. 7**C), although linear or curvilinear abnormal FDG uptake may be also seen on PET (**Fig. 7**D).

Multiplanar imaging also is important in the diagnosis of inflammatory disease and infections. Contrast-enhanced CT images can reveal the rim enhancement

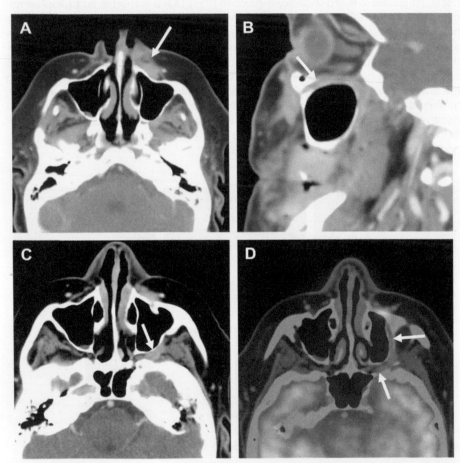

Fig. 7. Perineural tumor spread of recurrent squamous cell carcinoma of the left upper lip in a 65-year-old woman. Axial contrast-enhanced CT image (*A*) shows a recurrent tumor (*arrow*) obscuring the premaxillary fat. Sagittal CT image (*B*) shows thickening and enhancement of the infraorbital nerve and enlargement of the infraorbital canal (*arrow*). Axial contrast-enhanced CT image (*C*) at the infraorbital level demonstrates obliteration of fat within the left pterygopalatin fossa and pterygomaxillary fissure (*arrow*). PET/CT image (*D*) shows mildly increased FDG uptake along the course of the left infraorbital nerve and maxillary division of the trigeminal nerve (V2) (*arrows*).

seen in a peritonsillar abscess (**Fig. 8**). The presence of a sequestrum often seen in osteomyelitis and osteonecrosis can be easily noted in the multiplanar reconstructed CT images along with the laminated periosteal reaction (**Fig. 9**). Osteomyelitis with a thick periosteal reaction is seen as a lytic/sclerotic bony changes (**Fig. 10**). Osteoradionecrosis of the jaw after radiotherapy for oral cavity or oropharyngeal cancers is seen as an erosive and lytic process with no periosteal reaction (**Fig. 11**).

Maxillary sinusitis can be of odontogenic or nonodontogenic origin. The elevation and interruption of the sinus floor in relation to the maxillary molars can lead to mucosal thickening in the maxillary sinus (**Fig. 12**).

MULTIDECTOR ROW CT IN THE DIAGNOSIS OF TRAUMA

MDCT is the standard imaging modality to assess maxillofacial injury. Fractures after trauma of the maxillofacial region are complex due to involvement of several structures, including the maxillary, mandibular, zygomatic, temporal, frontal, ethmoid, and sphenoid bone. MDCT allows for high-quality MPR reformation and isotropic viewing, which helps in detecting both displaced and nondisplaced fractures.[18–20] CT is more sensitive than a panoramic image in diagnosing fractures of the angle, ramus, or condyles of the mandible (**Fig. 13**).[20] The mandible is a ringlike structure; therefore, a majority of mandibular fractures have been believed to be multifocal; however, recent studies used MDCT have revealed nearly half of the mandibular fractures can be unifocal.[21] Associated temporal bone fractures can be seen in 3% of the patients with mandibular fractures.[22]

EMERGING MULTIDETECTOR ROW CT TECHNIQUES IN MAXILLOFACIAL IMAGING
Perfusion Multidetector Row CT

In patients with head and neck malignancies, the pathologic processes are apparent before any radiographic anatomic changes. Functional imaging can distinguish disease by evaluating functional (blood and lymphatic flow), metabolic, and molecular

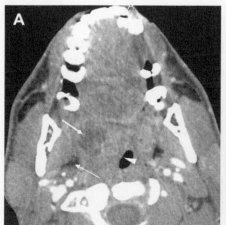
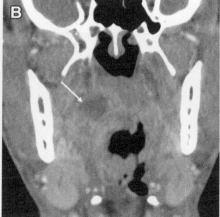

Fig. 8. Peritonsillar abscess in a 28-year-old man with dysphagia. Axial (*A*) and coronal (*B*) contrast-enhanced CT images show a rim-enhancing fluid collection (*arrows*) with swelling of the right palatine tonsil. Note narrowing of the oropharyngeal air way (*arrowhead*) and effacement of the parapharyngeal fat (*thin arrow*).

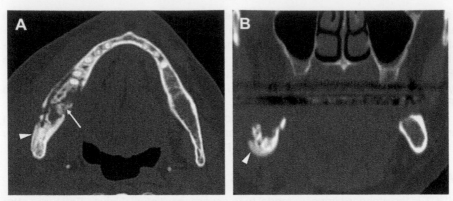

Fig. 9. Bisphosphonate-related osteonecrosis of the jaw in a 65-year-old woman. The patient has history of metastatic breast cancer treated with bisphosphonate several years ago. Axial (*A*) and coronal (*B*) CT images show mixed lytic and sclerotic changes and disruption of the lingual and buccal cortices of the right mandibular body with a sequestrum (*arrow*). Note periosteal reaction (*arrowheads*).

changes.[23,24] Perfusion MDCT, performed after intravenous bolus injection of contrast medium, permits functional evaluation of tissue vascularity and temporal tissue density changes. This aids in the diagnosis of lesion characterization, staging, tumor prognosis based on vascularity, and monitoring the response of various treatment regimens.[24]

The first-pass perfusion study images are acquired in the initial cine phase for a total of 40 seconds to 60 seconds, usually acquired every 1 second (deconvolution method). In permeability studies, a second phase is performed ranging from 2 minutes to 10 minutes.[24,25] One of the major concerns is the risk of increased dose of ionizing radiation, especially in patients who need serial studies to monitor treatment effects. Perfusion CT allows for quantification of the abnormal vasculature and thus permits assessment of tumor aggressiveness.[24,26]

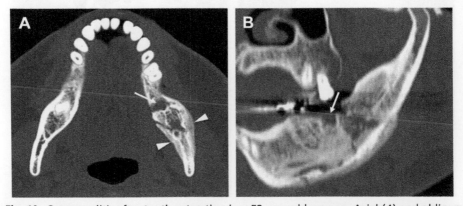

Fig. 10. Osteomyelitis after tooth extraction in a 52-year-old woman. Axial (*A*) and oblique sagittal (*B*) CT images show extraction socket (*arrows*), lysis of the trabecular bone with surrounding sclerosis. There is thick periosteal reaction along with the lingual and buccal surfaces of the left body and angle of the mandible (*arrowheads*).

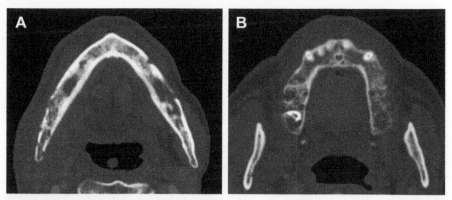

Fig. 11. Osteoradionecrosis in a 64-year-old man with a history of right tonsillar cancer treated with chemoradiotherapy 4 years ago. Axial CT images of the mandible (*A*) and maxillary alveolar ridge (*B*) show multifocal erosions of the cortex and lucencies in the cancellous bone bilaterally in both mandible and maxilla.

Dual-Energy CT

Dual-energy CT (DECT) scanners have 2 x-ray tubes allowing for simultaneous acquisition of images at 2 different energy levels, usually 80 kVp and 140 kVp.[27–30] The acquired data are reconstructed into low-energy and high-energy data sets, which can be combined to maximize contrast and minimize noise and leads to reduction in metal artifacts. Linear blending is one of the most common postprocessing DECT data and provides a blended image that closely resembles a standard single-energy image. Nonlinear blending algorithms consists of merging selective low-kVp and high-kVp data sets with several weighting factors within the same tissue.[29,31]

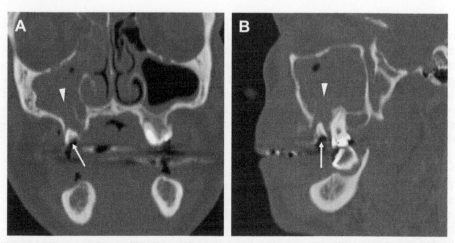

Fig. 12. Odontogenic maxillary sinusitis in a 52-year-old man. Coronal (*A*) and sagittal (*B*) CT images show mucosal thickening and opacification of the right maxillary sinus secondary to infected radicular cyst. Note carious defects of maxillary first molar (*arrows*), elevation and partial disappearing of the sinus floor (*arrowheads*).

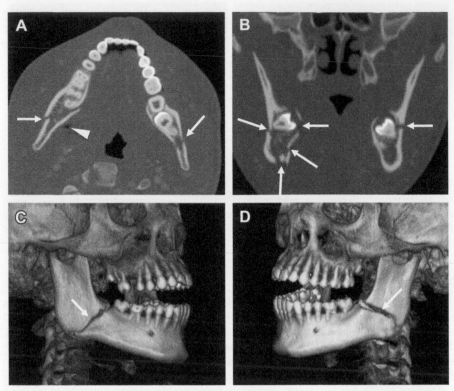

Fig. 13. Bilateral mandibular fractures in a 16-year-old man. Axial (*A*), coronal (*B*), and 3-D reconstructed (*C, D*) CT images show bilateral superior to inferior obliquely oriented comminuted fractures through the bilateral mandibular angles which involve the mandibular canal (*arrows*). Note the associated emphysema in the surrounding soft tissues (*arrowhead*).

DECT imaging allows for material differentiation and characterization by creating monochromatic energy images. Iodine-specific DECT images allow for iodine quantization and are better for estimating tumor invasion and involvement of lymph nodes. If the iodine concentration is known, it can be subtracted from mixed dataset to generate a virtual noncontrast image (**Fig. 14**). It can aid in differentiating between malignant and benign lymph nodes based on iodine concentration.[31] DECT aids to detect recurrent disease and discriminate it from benign post-treatment changes of the tissues. Similarly, a virtual noncalcium image can be generated, which allows for assessment of bone marrow edema.[27,31]

CT Texture Analysis

Texture analysis is a postprocessing technique that extracts information native to image data that is not apparent on visual inspection of images. These techniques ultimately provide a quantitative means of extracting image features that are useful for comparative analyses. In the past several years, CT texture analysis has been investigated in oncology imaging including head and neck cancers to predict human papillomavirus status,[32,33] which is important for treatment outcome. More recent study indicates CT texture analysis may be new biomarkers for advanced oncologic imaging in precision medicine and outcomes to treatment.[34–36]

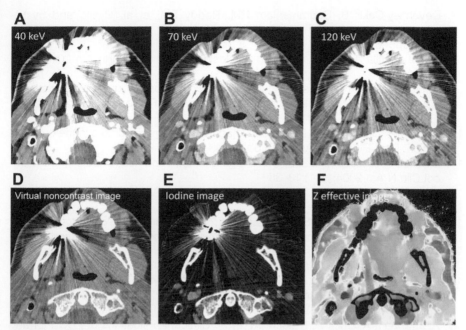

Fig. 14. DECT applications. (*A–C*) Virtual monochromatic image (VMI) reconstructions ([*A*] 40 keV; [*B*] 70 keV; [*C*] 120 keV). Increased attenuation of the vessel is obtained on lower-keV VMIs, closer to the k edge of iodine, at the expense of increased image noise. (*D*) Virtual noncontrast image almost completely eliminates high attenuation within the vessel on post-contrast CT. (*E*) Iodine image better depicts iodine-containing structures, such as vessels and enhancing lesions, and also can help reduce streak artifact. (*F*) Z effective image distinguishes different materials based on atomic number and may help distinguish different lesions. (*Courtesy of* Dr Kristine Mosier, Indiana University School of Medicine, Indianapolis, IN.)

SUMMARY

Multiplanar imaging with good soft tissue contrast and spatial resolution has contributed to the widespread use of MDCT in the diagnosis of head and neck lesions. The recent advances in MDCT technology will be an integrated anatomic and functional high-resolution scan with lower radiation doses, which will help in diagnosis of maxillofacial lesions and overall patient care.

REFERENCES

1. Prokop M. General principles of MDCT. Eur J Radiol 2003;45(Suppl 1):S4–10.
2. Mupparapu M, Nadeau C. Oral and maxillofacial imaging. Dent Clin North Am 2016;60(1):1–37.
3. Rogalla P, Kloeters C, Hein PA. CT technology overview: 64-slice and beyond. Radiol Clin North Am 2009;47(1):1–pp11.
4. Imhof H, Czerny C, Dirisamer A. Head and neck imaging with MDCT. Eur J Radiol 2003;45(Suppl 1):S23–31.
5. Rubin GD. 3-D imaging with MDCT. Eur J Radiol 2003;45(Suppl 1):S37–41.
6. Baum U, Greess H, Lell M, et al. Imaging of head and neck tumors—methods. Eur J Radiol 2000;33:153–60.

7. Devenney-Cakir B, Subramaniam RM, Reddy SM, et al. Cystic and cystic-appearing lesions of the mandible: review. AJR Am J Roentgenol 2011; 196(Suppl 6):WS66–77.

8. Gohel A, Villa A, Sakai O. Benign jaw lesions. Dent Clin North Am 2016;60(1): 125–41.

9. Dunfee BL, Sakai O, Pistey R, et al. Radiologic and pathologic characteristics of benign and malignant lesions of the mandible. Radiographics 2006;26(6): 1751–68.

10. Singer SR, Creanga AG. Diagnostic imaging of malignant tumors in the orofacial region. Dent Clin North Am 2016;60(1):143–65.

11. Alberico RA, Husain SH, Sirotkin I. Imaging in head and neck oncology. Surg Oncol Clin N Am 2004;13(1):13–35.

12. Rana RS, Wu JS, Eisenberg RL. Periosteal reaction. AJR Am J Roentgenol 2009; 193(4):W259–72.

13. Roh J-L, Yeo N-K, Kim JS, et al. Utility of 2-[18F] fluoro-2-deoxy-d-glucose positron emission tomography and positron emission tomography/computed tomography imaging in the preoperative staging of head and neck squamous cell carcinoma. Oral Oncol 2007;43(9):887–93.

14. Goel R, Moore W, Sumer B, et al. Clinical practice in PET/CT for the management of head and neck squamous cell cancer. AJR Am J Roentgenol 2017;209(2): 289–303.

15. Al-Ibraheem A, Buck A, Krause BJ, et al. Clinical applications of FDG PET and PET/CT in head and neck cancer. J Oncol 2009;2009:208725.

16. Kito S, Koga H, Kodama M, et al. Reflection of ^{18}F-FDG accumulation in the evaluation of the extent of periapical or periodontal inflammation. Oral Surg Oral Med Oral Pathol Oral Radiol 2012;114(6):e62–9.

17. Binmadi NO, Basile JR. Perineural invasion in oral squamous cell carcinoma: a discussion of significance and review of the literature. Oral Oncol 2011;47(11): 1005–10.

18. Badger D, Aygun N. Imaging of perineural spread in head and neck cancer. Radiol Clin North Am 2017;55(1):139–49.

19. Sung EK, Nadgir RN, Sakai O. Computed tomographic imaging in head and neck trauma: what the radiologist needs to know. Semin Roentgenol 2012;47(4):320–9.

20. Lo Casto A, Priolo GD, Garufi A, et al. Imaging evaluation of facial complex strut fractures. Semin Ultrasound CT MR 2012;33(5):396–409.

21. Ogura T, Kaneda S, Mori K, et al. Characterization of mandibular fractures using 64-slice multidetector CT. Dentomaxillofac Radiol 2012;41:392–5.

22. Buch K, Mottalib A, Nadgir RN, et al. Unifocal versus multifocal mandibular fractures and injury location. Emerg Radiol 2016;23(2):161–7.

23. Ogura I, Kaneda T, Sasaki Y, et al. Prevalence of temporal bone fractures in patients with mandibular fractures using multidetector-row CT. Clin Neuroradiol 2015;25(2):137–41.

24. Petralia G, Bonello L, Viotti S, et al. CT perfusion in oncology: how to do it. Cancer Imaging 2010;10(1):8–19.

25. Razek AA, Tawfik AM, Elsorogy LG, et al. Perfusion CT of head and neck cancer. Eur J Radiol 2014;83(3):537–44.

26. Preda L, Calloni SF, Moscatelli ME, et al. Role of CT perfusion in monitoring and prediction of response to therapy of head and neck squamous cell carcinoma. Biomed Res Int 2014;2014:917150.

27. Bisdas S, Baghi M, Smolarz A, et al. Quantitative measurements of perfusion and permeability of oropharyngeal and oral cavity cancer, recurrent disease, and

associated lymph nodes using first-pass contrast-enhanced computed tomography studies. Invest Radiol 2007;42(3):172–9.

28. Roele ED, Timmer VCML, Vaassen LAA, et al. Dual-energy CT in head and neck imaging. Curr Radiol Rep 2017;5(5):19.

29. Yamauchi H, Buehler M, Goodsitt MM, et al. Dual-energy CT-based differentiation of benign posttreatment changes from primary or recurrent malignancy of the head and neck: comparison of spectral hounsfield units at 40 and 70 keV and iodine concentration. AJR Am J Roentgenol 2016;206(3):580–7.

30. Vogl TJ, Schulz B, Bauer RW, et al. Dual-energy CT applications in head and neck imaging. AJR Am J Roentgenol 2012;199(Suppl 5):S34–9.

31. Kuno H, Sekiya K, Chapman MN, et al. Miscellaneous and emerging applications of dual-energy computed tomography for the evaluation of intracranial pathology. Neuroimaging Clin N Am 2017;27(3):411–42.

32. Ginat DT, Mayich M, Daftari-Besheli L, et al. Clinical applications of dual-energy CT in head and neck imaging. Eur Arch Otorhinolaryngol 2016;273(3):547–53.

33. Buch K, Fujita A, Li B, et al. Using texture analysis to determine human papillomavirus status of oropharyngeal squamous cell carcinomas on CT. AJNR Am J Neuroradiol 2015;36(7):1343–8.

34. Fujita A, Buch K, Li B, et al. Difference between HPV-positive and HPV-negative non-oropharyngeal head and neck cancer: texture analysis features on CT. J Comput Assist Tomogr 2016;40(1):43–7.

35. Kuno H, Qureshi MM, Chapman MN, et al. CT texture analysis potentially predicts local failure in head and neck squamous cell carcinoma treated with chemoradiotherapy. AJNR Am J Neuroradiol 2017. https://doi.org/10.3174/ajnr.A5407.

36. Becker M. CT texture analysis: defining and integrating new biomarkers for advanced oncologic imaging in precision medicine: a comment on "CT texture analysis potentially predicts wlocal failure in head and neck squamous cell carcinoma treated with chemoradiotherapy". AJNR Am J Neuroradiol 2017. https://doi.org/10.3174/ajnr.A5451.

MRI for Dental Applications

Husniye Demirturk Kocasarac, DDS, PhD[a],*, Hassem Geha, DDS, MDS[a],
Laurence R. Gaalaas, DDS, MS[b], Donald R. Nixdorf, DDS, MS[c]

KEYWORDS

- MRI • Dental MRI • UTE • SWIFT • ZTE • FLASH • Tooth • Jaw

KEY POINTS

- MRI is a well-developed medical imaging technology, being the imaging modality of choice for most soft tissue and functional imaging indications.
- The science and application of MRI continue to advance, with several recent developments having notable implications for the practice of dentistry.
- Although MRI has traditionally been considered prohibitively costly for use in routine dental practice, many of the recent technological advancements have the potential to greatly reduce the cost associated with manufacturing and operating an MRI scanner.

INTRODUCTION

Visualize an MRI scanner that is less expensive and designed to image a smaller field of view (FOV), like a knee, ankle, or wrist. Such anatomy-specific MRI scanners have been developed and are currently or soon to be available.[1] Facilitating this development is an MRI design shift away from using larger and more expensive magnets with excellent field homogeneity and toward accepting smaller, less homogeneous (or less perfect) magnetic fields produced by cheaper and smaller magnets. Image formation can remain feasible by computationally correcting for magnet inhomogeneity and technological advances in pulse sequences and coil design, allowing for MRI scanners to become even cheaper to manufacture.[1–3] Now, imagine optimizing these smaller FOV scanners to image teeth, the jaws, and face, and you have the design of an MRI scanner designed for dental use.

The physics of producing an image with magnetic resonance are more complex and quite different from computed tomography (CT) or cone beam computed tomography

Disclosure: The authors have nothing to disclose.
[a] Division of Oral and Maxillofacial Radiology, Department of Comprehensive Dentistry, University of Texas Health San Antonio, 7703 Floyd Curl Drive, San Antonio, TX 78229, USA;
[b] Oral and Maxillofacial Radiology, Division of Oral Medicine, Diagnosis and Radiology, Department of Diagnostic and Biological Sciences, School of Dentistry, University of Minnesota, 7-536 Moos Tower, 515 Delaware Street Southeast, Minneapolis, MN 55455, USA; [c] Division of TMD and Orofacial Pain, Department of Diagnostic and Biological Sciences, School of Dentistry, University of Minnesota, 6-320 Moos Tower, 515 Delaware Street SE, Minneapolis, MN 55455, USA
* Corresponding author.
E-mail address: demirturk@uthscsa.edu

Dent Clin N Am 62 (2018) 467–480
https://doi.org/10.1016/j.cden.2018.03.006
0011-8532/18/© 2018 Elsevier Inc. All rights reserved.

dental.theclinics.com

(CBCT) using radiograph. Consequently, MRI has considerably more opportunity for producing useful depictions of human tissues. With the development of dental and face-specific MRI coils, plus the freedom found in sequence design and image processing, researchers can feasibly develop custom techniques to address any number of dental imaging indications: anatomic characterization of hard tissues including bone and teeth for "routine" dental indications like implant placement, caries detection, and fracture detection; anatomic and functional characterization of soft tissues, including periodontal/periapical inflammation, muscle and nerves to characterize neural and pain disorders, and pathologic tissue characterization to diagnose neoplasms and dysplasia without a surgical biopsy; blood flow imaging in both bulk and perfusion forms to assess tissue viability/inflammatory status; and finally, spectroscopy to provide molecular profiles of tissue. Related technological advances in pulse sequence design will likely lead us into uncharted knowledge about normal dental anatomy and physiology as well as pathology and pathophysiology.

In this article, the authors provide a brief overview of the use of conventional MRI techniques applied to dental indications, discuss relevant MRI physics in the various steps of image formation, and highlight recent hardware and software technical developments that contribute to (1) the cost/size of MRI decreasing significantly, allowing use in the typical dental clinic, and (2) the facilitation of very specific dental imaging applications that will solve clinical problems.

ESTABLISHED MRI TECHNIQUES APPLIED TO DENTAL INDICATIONS

The first MRI was acquired by Lauterbur in 1973.[4] With the evolution of the commercial medical MRI in the 1980s, several applications were performed in medical imaging (ie, cardiac, abdominal, cranial MRI).[5] Broadly, in medicine, MRI is fast outpacing any other modality for in vivo displaying of soft tissues and function in the human body without any invasive procedure and ionizing radiation.[6] Because of the inability of conventional MRI to image hard tissues, conventional MRI techniques in dentistry have been mostly used for soft tissue imaging, including the temporomandibular joints (TMJ), soft tissues, tumors, salivary glands, and maxillary sinuses.[7] Currently, TMJ imaging comprises the vast majority of dedicated MRI imaging for clinical dental indications with diagnostic accuracy of joint characterization and disc localization high enough that the modality is considered the gold standard.[8–10]

Other applications of MRI for dental indications include caries detection, pulpal/periapical disease characterization, and some efforts at inferior alveolar nerve identification. These efforts have been limited largely to research/experimental reports and have not been adopted clinically. The use of MRI to visualize dental caries was first described by van Luijk in 1981[11] with later studies stating that the caries under a restoration, which cannot be easily seen on a conventional radiograph, may be detected by MRI in the future.[5]

MRI for pulpal and periapical disease characterization appears promising with successful imaging of pulp morphology, visualization of pulpitis/pulp vitality, and assessment of pulpal regeneration.[12] MRI has demonstrated some experimental utility in identifying the location of the mandibular nerve in the context of mandibular dental implant and surgery planning.[13,14]

A BRIEF OVERVIEW OF MRI PHYSICS AND STEPWISE DESCRIPTION OF HOW AN MRI IS OBTAINED

Before recent developments in MRI research specific to dental imaging and as a matter of review are discussed, the following is a brief discussion of how diagnostic images are obtained using MRI.

Step 1. Place a Patient in a Large Magnet

Every single hydrogen (hydrogen-1) nucleus in a patient or object otherwise has its own tiny magnetic field. Hydrogen nuclei (mostly water) in aggregate have essentially randomly oriented magnetic fields, but when placed in a strong magnetic field, they align and incur precession (resonance) with the magnetic field like tiny spinning toy tops. Accordingly, when a patient or object is placed in an MRI magnetic field, every hydrogen nucleus aligns and incurs precession in the direction of the magnetic field, the first step in enabling capture of a MR image. Generally, MRI units are measured by the strength of the magnet with units of Tesla, where 1 T is the equivalent of 20,000 times the magnetic field strength of Earth. The vast majority of clinical MRI scanners in use today are either 1.5 T or 3 T for human procedures.[6]

Step 2. Use a Transmitting Radiofrequency Coil to Apply a Radiofrequency Pulse to the Patient in the Magnet

With the application of a radiofrequency (RF) pulse to the patient in the magnet, all of the patient's hydrogen nuclei realign their direction of precession to the direction of a RF pulse. Transmitting RF coils are typically built into the larger body of the physical MRI unit, with the magnet. The RF pulse is left on for variable amounts of time to initiate different degrees of resonance or realignment with the RF pulse. During realignment, all of the hydrogen nuclei absorb some amount of energy and create a new, tiny magnetic field in alignment with the applied RF pulse. This degree of energy input can be deliberately applied in order to emphasize or deemphasize various tissue types that otherwise can overall overwhelm aspects of an MRI image. Fat-suppressed images are one common example of this technique, in which the proper amount of RF energy applied later on results in minimal or zero contribution of fat to the image allowing better visualization of adjacent tissues of interest.[15,16] Similarly, fluid attenuated inversion recovery eliminates high signals seen from fluid/water and is used to detect parenchymal edema without the glaringly high signal from cerebrospinal fluid.[17–19]

Step 3. Stop the Radiofrequency Pulse and Use a Receiving Radiofrequency Coil to Collect and Record Radiofrequency Energy Released by the Hydrogen Nuclei as They Realign Back to the Original Magnet Field of the MRI Unit

A receiving coil used to collect and record the RF energy released by the patient may be the same coil as the transmitting coil (typically built into the scanner body), or it could be a separate receiving-only coil designed for imaging specific anatomic regions. These coils are commonly called "surface" coils because they are separate from the larger MRI physical unit, and they are applied close to the surface of the patient's anatomy to be imaged.

When hydrogen nuclei "relax" back to precession in alignment with the primary magnetic field of the unit, they do so with primarily 2 characteristic properties: T1 and T2. T1, or spin-lattice relaxation time, refers to an average time a group of hydrogen nuclei relax back to their initial energy level before the RF pulse. T2, or spin-spin relaxation time, refers to an average time a group of hydrogen nuclei having been subject to an applied RF pulse loses the tiny magnetic field created in alignment with that RF pulse. In practice, T1 sequences are common images in any MRI evaluation and are usually used as "anatomic" images.[20,21] Based on both the environment surrounding hydrogen nuclei (based largely on tissue type) and the overall concentration of hydrogen nuclei (also based largely on tissue type), different tissues have different T1 and T2 properties. The amount of T1 and T2 signal can be converted into pixel grayscale value once reconstructed. In pure T1-weighted images, fatty tissue demonstrates typically a high signal (bright), whereas muscles and other soft tissues demonstrate intermediate signal intensity (gray), and fluid demonstrates a low signal (black).

As discussed earlier, a fat-suppressed T1-weighted image is a variation of a T1 sequence where the bright signal from fat is cleverly eliminated (suppressed) for detection of other tissue's signals that can be obstructed by the fat signal.[15,16] In a contrast-enhanced T1-weighted image, a gadolinium-based contrast agent is injected intravenously, and scans are obtained a few minutes after administration. The gadolinium acts to shorten both T1 and T2 properties, thereby increasing tissue signal and ultimately image brightness. Because the contrast agent is applied intravenously, vascular structures and any pathologic condition with increased vascularity appear brighter on the MRI image. Frequently, postcontrast T1 sequences are also fat suppressed to make them easier to interpret.[22] T2 sequences are also common images in any MRI evaluation and are usually used as simplified "functional" or "pathologic" images because in many pathologic conditions, the water content increases, leading to an increase in the signal of those pathologic tissues.[20,21]

Proton density images represent an "overall" density of hydrogen in the patient with an image that is not biased or weighted to either T1 or T2 character. Proton density images are commonly used for brain imaging and also are excellent for TMJ imaging because they offer excellent signal distinction between fluid, hyaline cartilage, and fibrocartilage.[23,24] Diffusion-weighted imaging assesses the ease with which water molecules move around within a tissue and give insights into cellularity, cell swelling, and edema.[25,26]

Conventional MRI cannot easily show hard tissues, including bone and teeth, because of the low concentration of hydrogen protons that contribute to the magnetization, and also because of extremely fast T2 relaxation times not detectable with conventional techniques.[27] In other words, the signal from mineralized dental tissues decays faster than signal of liquids before MRI signal is detected. This phenomenon causes minimal or no image intensity (black image) MR images.[27]

MRI has an obvious advantage in the lack of use of ionizing radiation and associated added risk of cancer development to the patient; however, it should be noted that the presence of a strong magnetic field can affect ferromagnetic metals in the vicinity of the magnet. Therefore, MRI is typically not used for patients with cardiac pacemakers, implantable defibrillators, artificial heart valves, cerebral aneurysm clips, or ferrous foreign bodies in the eye.[8]

Technical developments enabling dental-specific MRI

There are several required main components to successfully image a patient or object with MRI: a strong magnet, body or surface coils, gradient coils, a pulse sequence, and software for digitized image reconstruction/manipulation/display. The authors describe these components along with recent technical developments they think will enable the construction of less expensive and dental-specific MRI units.

THE MAGNET

The largest component of a typical MRI scanner is the magnet itself, which is in essence a large insulated vessel containing wire windings and cryogen (ie, liquid helium) to enable a superconducting magnet. The manufacturing process for magnets with a small bore size requires less wire and cryogen and is therefore smaller, lighter, and cheaper. These smaller magnets facilitate the development of scanners that are dedicated in their purpose, such as dedicated head, knee, wrist, breast, or small animal imaging. This transition of large, whole-body MRI scanners to smaller, dedicated-purpose MRI scanners is similar to the development of a dental CBCT scanner from a multipurpose medical CT scanner.

Furthermore, the advent of high-temperature superconducting wire has eliminated the need for cryogens, which is expensive to purchase and bulky to use because of the required insulation and the need to pressurize the container that houses the windings.[28] These magnets are "plug in the wall" powered, with the only remaining major barrier to development the cost of manufacturing high-temperature superconducting material in continuous lengths needed for MRI use. An alternative approach to avoiding the use of cryogens is to use rare earth magnets, which have all the same benefits as high-temperature superconducting wiring but also have a high cost.[29] Rare earth magnets are also disadvantaged by their inability to achieve strong magnetic fields, such as 1.5 T, a minimum standard for obtaining high-quality images. The combinations of anatomy-specific scanners and scanners that avoid the use of cryogens result in systems greatly reduced in size, weight, and complexity, all requirements needed to realize the development of point-of-care dental MRI scanners. The potential development of a commercial market plus mass production of high-temperature superconducting wire will allow for a reduction in cost of manufacturing, further reducing overall costs.

BODY AND SURFACE COILS

Clinical MRI scanners are built with large RF coils within the bore of the scanner to transmit radio waves that energize the tissue being imaged. These RF coils are typically referred to as body coils, because they are built to energize the entire body, regardless of the anatomy being imaged. To record the RF signal released by the patient, anatomy-specific receiver or surface coils are placed adjacent to the anatomy being imaged. Per the discussion earlier, MRI scanners that are anatomy specific, such as a head-only scanner, reduce the need for these large body coils and associated cost. An alternative approach is to use transceiver coils that both transmit and receive the RF signal, thus eliminating the need for body coils altogether.[3] Because a coil acts as an antenna by detecting the signal emitted from the patient, the closer distance the coil is to the anatomy of interest to be imaged results in a greater amount of detectable signal from the tissue of interest. Consequently, designing coils to be anatomy specific allows for a smaller FOV to be used, and it results in the ability to decrease the voxel dimensions, thus increasing the capacity to obtain higher resolution images (**Figs. 1** and **2**).[30] The acquisition of high-resolution images is critical for dentistry, because visualization of small alterations in anatomy is commonly clinically significant. This approach has been used for dental applications, such as the extraoral approach of obtaining a close fit of the coil over the face,[31,32] and the intraoral approaches of placing the coil adjacent to the teeth (like a periapical film)[30] or in the orthogonal plane (like an occlusal film).[33] To improve comfort and usability, coils that transmit signal to the scanner wirelessly have been developed (**Figs. 3** and **4**).[34] It is hoped that the development of coils specific to teeth and supporting structures will enable FOVs that image not only teeth effectively but also the surrounding periodontium and alveolar bone.[33]

GRADIENT COILS

Gradient coils are located in the body of the magnet proper. The function of these coils is to impart a small change or gradient within the main magnetic field in each of the 3 dimensions of the patient, referred to as x-, y-, and z-directions. While the magnet is scanning, these gradient coils will be used to rapidly alter the local magnetic field, with

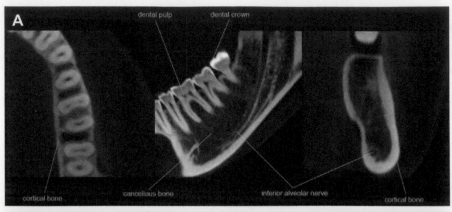

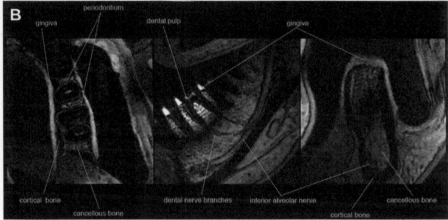

Fig. 1. (*B*) Axial (*left*), sagittal (*middle*), and transverse (*right*) cross-sections of FLASH MRI of the lower jaw acquired in vivo with an intraoral coil that was inductively coupled to a small loop coil at 3 T with the following parameters: 250 μm² × 500 μm resolution, 64 mm × 64 mm × 28 mm FOV, acquisition time 3:57 minutes. (*A*) Axial (*left*), sagittal (*middle*), and transverse (*right*) cross-sections of in vivo cone beam CT of the lower jaw (3D Accuitomo 170, Morita, Japan; nominal resolution, 250 μm, 90 kV, 201 images). (*From* Flügge T, Hövener JB, Ludwig U, et al. Magnetic resonance imaging of intraoral hard and soft tissues using an intraoral coil and FLASH sequences. Eur Radiol 2016;26:4621; with permission.)

larger gradients producing a greater ability to record spatial information. The rapid changes in gradients are responsible for producing the noise associated with MRI scanning, with some pulse sequences demanding fast and large gradient changes and associated noise (eg, functional MRI). A notable advantage of sweep imaging with Fourier transformation (SWIFT), a relatively new pulse sequence that has shown success at imaging hard tissue of teeth and bones, is relatively little demand on gradient coil changes and associated low noise/improved comfort for the patient.[27]

PULSE SEQUENCES

A pulse sequence is the code that instructs the MRI scanner in how to image the patient, similar to how software instructs a computer how to operate. Over time, new pulse sequences are developed to address new approaches to imaging, and clinically

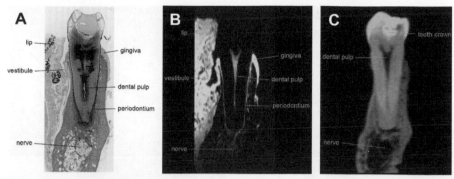

Fig. 2. (*A*) Histologic section through the second premolar in the left mandible of an ex vivo human specimen. (*B*) Section through the MRI of the tooth with identical visible structures. (*C*) Section through CBCT image of the ex vivo human specimen with fewer visible structures. (*From* Flügge T, Hövener JB, Ludwig U, et al. Magnetic resonance imaging of intraoral hard and soft tissues using an intraoral coil and FLASH sequences. Eur Radiol 2016;26:4619; with permission.)

robust ones are continuously updated. Also similar to computer software, matching the software (ie, pulse sequence) and the hardware (ie, magnet and coil) with each other is critical to get maximal production and efficiency for a given MRI scanner. The pulse sequence developments that are allowing the visualization of densely calcified tissue (eg, dentin, enamel, bone) are referred to as short T2, because they allow for capture of the rapidly decaying T2 signal inherent to hard tissues. SWIFT, ultrashort echo time (UTE), and zero echo time (ZTE) are all examples of relatively newly developed short T2 pulse sequences with efficacy in imaging hard tissue.

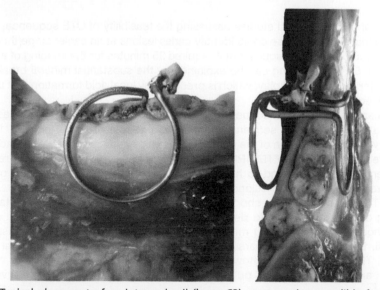

Fig. 3. Typical placement of an intraoral coil (here: C2) on a porcine mandible for ex vivo MRI. (*From* Ludwig U, Eisenbeiss A-K, Scheifele C, et al. Dental MRI using wireless intraoral coils. Sci Rep 2016;6:23301. This work is licensed under a Creative Commons Attribution 4.0 International License, Available at: http://creativecommons.org/licenses/by/4.0/.)

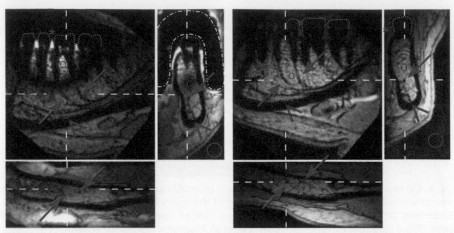

Fig. 4. In vivo dental MRI of a mandible acquired with (*Left*) and without (*Right*) intraoral coil C3 in conjunction with a 4-cm loop coil. Orthogonal slices were reconstructed from a 3D-FLASH MRI that was acquired in 3:57 minutes at 3 T at a resolution of 250 μm³ × 250 μm³ × 500 μm³. Note that the intraoral coil enhanced the signal of the inter-dental gingiva (*asterisk*) and pulp strongly and caused a signal hypointensity at the roots. Both configurations nicely depicted the inferior alveolar nerve and its branches to the apices of the teeth (rami dentales) as indicated by arrows and wedges, respectively. Dashed lines indicate the position of the reconstructed slices; dotted lines indicate the crowns of the teeth, and dash-dot lines indicate the position of the intraoral coil. The regions where the signal and noise was measured are indicated by asterisks (gingiva) and circless. (*From* Ludwig U, Eisenbeiss A-K, Scheifele C, et al. Dental MRI using wireless intraoral coils. Sci Rep 2016;6:23301. This work is licensed under a Creative Commons Attribution 4.0 International License, Available at: http://creativecommons.org/licenses/by/4.0/.)

In one of the first clinical studies assessing the feasibility of UTE sequence, it was reported that UTE sequence could identify caries lesions at an earlier stage than conventional radiograph techniques, but it required 25 minutes for the imaging of a single tooth (**Fig. 5**).[35] This finding can be explained by the substantial mineral breakdown required for radiograph display, which is preceded by local acid formation that is likely to be detected with MRI.[36]

The feasibility of the ZTE sequence to assess tooth tissue components has been investigated in vitro. ZTE sequence, applied to extracted human teeth at 11.7 T, yielded very good depiction of the mineralized dentine and enamel layers. In addition, compared with micro-CT, ZTE MRI was found to be less sensitive to artifacts resulted from dental restorations and to have superior sensitivity for the detection of early demineralization and caries lesions (**Fig. 6**).[36]

SWIFT sequence, with a short TE using intraoral coil, enabled simultaneous imaging of both soft and hard dental tissues with a high resolution and in a relatively short scanning time (10 minutes). Despite soft tissues not being displayed in detail, this technique appears to be promising and practical for clinical applications. The sequence also showed promise in determining the extent of carious lesions and the status of pulpal tissue, whether reversible or irreversible pulpitis.[27]

In a recent study performed by using SWIFT sequence, with a cable-bound intraoral coil, teeth of the upper and lower jaw were displayed in vivo in 4.5 minutes. It was also stated that the first MRI panoramic images at such high nominal resolution (0.3 mm³)

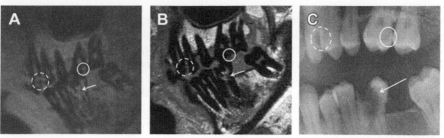

Fig. 5. Appearance of an initial caries (CIII, *circle*), secondary caries in the proximity of an amalgam filling (CI, *dashed circle*), and progressed caries lesion with related breakdown of the enamel and dentin layer (CI, *arrow*) in UTE (*A*), spin echo (*B*), and XR (*C*). (*From* Bracher AK, Hofmann C, Bornstedt A, et al. Feasibility of ultra-short echo time (UTE) magnetic resonance imaging for identification of carious lesions. Magn Reson Med 2011;66(2):542; with permission.)

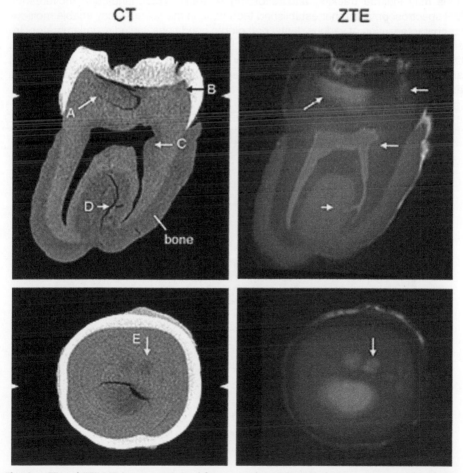

Fig. 6. μCT and ZTE MR images acquired from a molar with caries lesions. Some residual bone attached to the teeth is visible. Occlusal demineralized lesion (*arrows A, B*), Halo effect around the pulp (*arrow C*), the fissures visible with mCT inside the dentine (*arrow D*), demineralized lesions (*arrow E*). (*From* Weiger M, Pruessmann KP, Bracher AK, et al. High-resolution ZTE imaging of human teeth. NMR Biomed 2012;25(10):1148; with permission.)

were achieved. With this approach, the periapical region, alveolar bone, and inferior alveolar nerve were not visualized (**Fig. 7**).[33]

One interesting attribute of the use of T2-weighted images is improved visualization of water content in hard and soft tissue. One study demonstrated the use T2 sequences in identifying cracks in teeth, specifically the contrast between relatively water-poor dental hard tissue and the small abnormality of a crack that contains more water content. As verified by micro-CT, fractures smaller than the voxel size of the MRI scan were visualized simply because of overwhelming signal from water content in the crack.[37]

More excitingly, 4D imaging can be used to measure blood flow in tissue. This technique is established in medicine for assessing perfusion in brains injured from a stroke.[38] Translating this approach to dental applications, emerging data suggest that blood flow in teeth can be measured, a development that may mark drastically improved assessment of tooth pulp vitality and disease status (**Fig. 8**). Other indications may include tracking and recording real-time TMJ/mandibular movements. MR spectroscopy, another established technique in medicine,[39] may enable molecular characterization of various dental pathologic conditions, including inflammatory lesions, dysplasia, neoplasms, as well as characterization of normal tissue function. Diffusion tensor imaging, a relatively new variation of diffusion-weighted imaging, and other related sequences may represent an avenue of future mandibular nerve anatomic and functional imaging.[40,41]

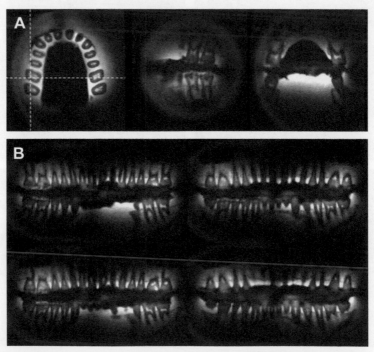

Fig. 7. Three selected orthogonal slices (*A*) and selected panoramic slices (*B*) of a 3D SWIFT image obtained using the transverse components of the B1 field. (*From* Idiyatullin D, Corum CA, Nixdorf DR, et al. Intraoral approach for imaging teeth using the transverse B1 field components of an occlusally oriented loop coil. Magn Reson Med 2014;72(1):164; with permission.)

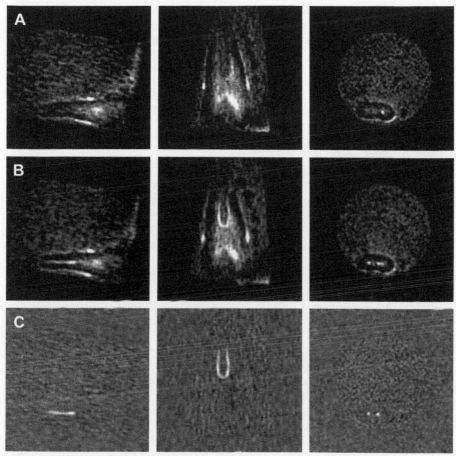

Fig. 8. (*A*) SWIFT MRI with blood-inflow saturation technique orthogonal sections of an extracted tooth with simulated fluid flow in the pulp chamber at 0.75 cm/s. (*B*) Similar orthogonal images with flow adjusted to 12 cm/s. (*C*) Image subtraction of 12 cm/s flow versus no flow demonstrating visualization of active fluid flow. These images are taken from unpublished data, 2017 performed by authors Nixdorf DR and Gaalaas L.

COMPUTING POWER AND IMAGE RECONSTRUCTION

In recent years, the computing power of personal computers built and priced for the consumer market have become adequate in handling most of the image reconstruction needs, thus decreasing the cost of MRI scanning systems. Only a few years ago MRI systems required expensive and purpose-built computer hardware to take the raw signals from the scanner and construct images from them. In addition, the algorithms for image reconstruction have improved, resulting in drastic reductions in time required to obtain useable images.

SUMMARY

In the last several years, major technological advancements involving multiple components of MRI have occurred. Together, they are enabling the hardware of MRI to become smaller, less complicated, cheaper, and tailored to acquiring images of teeth and supporting structures. Research investigating the clinical utility of this technology to address problems in dentistry is just now initiating, and consequently, the application of MRI in dentistry is feasible with potential yet to be explored.

REFERENCES

1. Sutter R, Tresch F, Buck FM, et al. Is dedicated extremity 1.5-T MRI equivalent to standard large-bore 1.5-T MRI for foot and knee examinations? AJR Am J Roentgenol 2014;203(6):1293–302.
2. Snyder AL, Corum CA, Moeller S, et al. MRI by steering resonance through space. Magn Reson Med 2014;72(1):49–58.
3. Sohn SM, Vaughan JT, Lagore RL, et al. In vivo MR imaging with simultaneous RF transmission and reception. Magn Reson Med 2016;76(6):1932–8.
4. Scherzinger AL, Hendee WR. Basic principles of magnetic resonance imaging–an update. The Western journal of medicine 1985;143(6):782–92.
5. Tymofiyeva O, Boldt J, Rottner K, et al. High-resolution 3D magnetic resonance imaging and quantification of carious lesions and dental pulp in vivo. MAGMA 2009;22(6):365–74.
6. Shah N, Bansal N, Logani A. Recent advances in imaging technologies in dentistry. World J Radiol 2014;6(10):794–807.
7. Tymofiyeva O, Rottner K, Jakob PM, et al. Three-dimensional localization of impacted teeth using magnetic resonance imaging. Clin Oral Investig 2010; 14(2):169–76.
8. Niraj LK, Patthi B, Singla A, et al. MRI in dentistry- a future towards radiation free imaging - systematic review. J Clin Diagn Res 2016;10(10):ZE14–9.
9. Suenaga S, Nagayama K, Nagasawa T, et al. The usefulness of diagnostic imaging for the assessment of pain symptoms in temporomandibular disorders. Jpn Dent Sci Rev 2016;52(4):93–106.
10. Boeddinghaus R, Whyte A. Trends in maxillofacial imaging. Clin Radiol 2018; 73(1):4–18.
11. van Luijk JA. NMR: dental imaging without x-rays? Oral Surg Oral Med Oral Pathol 1981;52(3):321–4.
12. Ariji Y, Ariji E, Nakashima M, et al. Magnetic resonance imaging in endodontics: a literature review. Oral Radiol 2017. https://doi.org/10.1007/s11282-017-0301-0.
13. Chau A. Comparison between the use of magnetic resonance imaging and conebeam computed tomography for mandibular nerve identification. Clin Oral Implants Res 2012;23(2):253–6.
14. Eggers G, Rieker M, Fiebach J, et al. Geometric accuracy of magnetic resonance imaging of the mandibular nerve. Dentomaxillofac Radiol 2005;34(5):285–91.
15. Bydder GM, Hajnal JV, Young IR. MRI: use of the inversion recovery pulse sequence. Clin Radiol 1998;53(3):159–76.
16. Lahrech H, Briguet A, Graveron-Demilly D, et al. Modified stimulated echo sequence for elimination of signals from stationary spins in MRI. Magn Reson Med 1987;5(2):196–200.
17. Lenclos N, Oppenheim C, Dormont D, et al. MRI of drug-resistant epilepsies: contribution of FLAIR sequence in a series of 150 patients. J Neuroradiol 2000; 27(3):164–72 [in French].
18. Textor HJ, Flacke S, Pauleit D. Acute spinal epidural hematoma–comments on MRI diagnosis using fluid-attenuated inversion recovery sequence (FLAIR). Rofo 1999;170(2):231–2 [in German].

19. Morioka T, Nishio S, Mihara F, et al. Efficacy of the fluid attenuated inversion recovery (FLAIR) sequence of MRI as a preoperative diagnosis of hippocampal sclerosis. No Shinkei Geka 1998;26(2):143–50 [in Japanese].

20. Mitchell MR, Tarr RW, Conturo TE, et al. Spin echo technique selection: basic principles for choosing MRI pulse sequence timing intervals. Radiographics 1986;6(2):245–60.

21. Mitchell MR, Conturo TE, Gruber TJ, et al. AUR Memorial Award. Two computer models for selection of optimal magnetic resonance imaging (MRI) pulse sequence timing. Invest Radiol 1984;19(5):350–60.

22. Goddard P, Waring J, Case A, et al. The STIR sequence in MRI of neoplastic lesions. Bristol Med Chir J (1963) 1988;103(2):26.

23. Tokuda O, Harada Y, Shiraishi G, et al. MRI of the anatomical structures of the knee: the proton density-weighted fast spin-echo sequence vs the proton density-weighted fast-recovery fast spin-echo sequence. Br J Radiol 2012; 85(1017):e686–93.

24. Lufkin RB, Keen R, Rhodes M, et al. MRI simulator for instruction in pulse-sequence selection. AJR Am J Roentgenol 1986;147(1):199–202.

25. Merboldt KD, Bruhn H, Frahm J, et al. MRI of "diffusion" in the human brain: new results using a modified CE-FAST sequence. Magn Reson Med 1989;9(3):423–9.

26. Genovese E, Cani A, Rizzo S, et al. Comparison between MRI with spin-echo echo-planar diffusion-weighted sequence (DWI) and histology in the diagnosis of soft-tissue tumours. Radiol Med 2011;116(4):644–56.

27. Idiyatullin D, Corum C, Moeller S, et al. Dental magnetic resonance imaging: making the invisible visible. J endodontics 2011;37(6):745–52.

28. Piao R, Iguchi S, Hamada M, et al. High resolution NMR measurements using a 400MHz NMR with an (RE)Ba2Cu3O7-x high-temperature superconducting inner coil: towards a compact super-high-field NMR. J Magn Reson 2016;263:164–71.

29. Besheer A, Caysa H, Metz H, et al. Benchtop-MRI for in vivo imaging using a macromolecular contrast agent based on hydroxyethyl starch (HES). Int J Pharm 2011;417(1–2):196–203.

30. Flugge T, Hovener JB, Ludwig U, et al. Magnetic resonance imaging of intraoral hard and soft tissues using an intraoral coil and FLASH sequences. Eur Radiol 2016;26(12):4616–23.

31. Prager M, Heiland S, Gareis D, et al. Dental MRI using a dedicated RF-coil at 3 Tesla. J Craniomaxillofac Surg 2015;43(10):2175–82.

32. Sedlacik J, Kutzner D, Khokale A, et al. Optimized 14 + 1 receive coil array and position system for 3D high-resolution MRI of dental and maxillomandibular structures. Dentomaxillofac Radiol 2016;45(1):20150177.

33. Idiyatullin D, Corum CA, Nixdorf DR, et al. Intraoral approach for imaging teeth using the transverse B1 field components of an occlusally oriented loop coil. Magn Reson Med 2014;72(1):160–5.

34. Ludwig U, Eisenbeiss AK, Scheifele C, et al. Dental MRI using wireless intraoral coils. Sci Rep 2016;6:23301.

35. Bracher AK, Hofmann C, Bornstedt A, et al. Feasibility of ultra-short echo time (UTE) magnetic resonance imaging for identification of carious lesions. Magn Reson Med 2011;66(2):538–45.

36. Weiger M, Pruessmann KP, Bracher AK, et al. High-resolution ZTE imaging of human teeth. NMR Biomed 2012;25(10):1144–51.

37. Idiyatullin D, Garwood M, Gaalaas L, et al. Role of MRI for detecting micro cracks in teeth. Dentomaxillofac Radiol 2016;45(7):20160150.

38. Burris NS, Hope MD. 4D flow MRI applications for aortic disease. Magn Reson Imaging Clin N Am 2015;23(1):15–23.
39. Liu Y, Gu Y, Yu X. Assessing tissue metabolism by phosphorous-31 magnetic resonance spectroscopy and imaging: a methodology review. Quant Imaging Med Surg 2017;7(6):707–26.
40. Arab A, Wojna-Pelczar A, Khairnar A, et al. Principles of diffusion kurtosis imaging and its role in early diagnosis of neurodegenerative disorders. Brain Res Bull 2018;139:91–8.
41. Terumitsu M, Matsuzawa H, Seo K, et al. High-contrast high-resolution imaging of posttraumatic mandibular nerve by 3DAC-PROPELLER magnetic resonance imaging: correlation with the severity of sensory disturbance. Oral Surg Oral Med Oral Pathol Oral Radiol 2017;124(1):85–94.

Ultrasound in Dentistry
Toward a Future of Radiation-Free Imaging

Husniye Demirturk Kocasarac, DDS, PhD[a],*, Christos Angelopoulos, DDS, MS[b]

KEYWORDS

- Ultrasonography • Diagnostic ultrasound • Dentistry • Jaw • Diagnosis
- Diagnostic imaging • Pathologic conditions

KEY POINTS

- Ultrasonography (US) is a non-invasive, non-ionizing, inexpensive and painless imaging tool, therefore, it can be performed as much as needed in a very short time.
- Well-known features of US are fast, cost-effective, reproducible, real time and simultaneous imaging of both hard and soft tissue, and easy tolerability by patient.
- US has been used to discover its capability to identify caries lesions, tooth fractures, soft tissue lesions, periodontal bony defects, maxillofacial fractures, and temporomandibular disorders.

REVIEW OF THE LITERATURE

Ultrasound refers to oscillating sounds with frequencies of 2 to 20 MHz, which is beyond the upper limit that humans can hear. Ultrasonography (US), also known as real-time echography or sonography, is an imaging technique based on the propagation and reflection of ultrasound waves in the tissues. The transducer includes an electrically stimulating piezoelectric crystal that converts electrical impulses to high-frequency sound waves, which are transmitted into the tissues being examined. As this sound passes through tissues with different acoustic impedances (ie, blood and muscle), part of it is absorbed within the medium; another part of it continues to penetrate and travel through the tissues. Finally, a portion of the sound is reflected back to the transducer and smaller portions of it may be scattered and lost. Echo is the part of the sound wave that is reflected back toward the surface of the body. The reflected echoes are collected by the transducer and reconverted into electrical impulses, amplified, processed, and displayed as grayscale images on a computer screen.[1]

Generally, ultrasound with frequencies between 3 MHz and 12 MHz is used in dentistry.[2] The most commonly used dental display modes are amplitude mode

Disclosure: The authors have nothing to disclose.
[a] Division of Oral and Maxillofacial Radiology, Department of Comprehensive Dentistry, UT Health San Antonio, 7703 Floyd Curl Drive, San Antonio, TX 78229, USA; [b] Aristotle University of Thessaloniki, Greece and Columbia University, College of Dental Medicine, Greece
* Corresponding author.
E-mail address: demirturk@uthscsa.edu

Dent Clin N Am 62 (2018) 481–489
https://doi.org/10.1016/j.cden.2018.03.007
0011-8532/18/© 2018 Elsevier Inc. All rights reserved.

dental.theclinics.com

(A-mode) and brightness mode (B-mode).[3] A-mode ultrasound is the most basic display mode after plotting the radiofrequency (RF) signal and was used often in early US. It uses a single crystal to generate a 1-dimensional image with the echo amplitude, displayed vertically, and the echo time, displayed horizontally. Currently, a standard screen image created by US machines is in B-mode. B-mode ultrasound images can be produced by moving an ultrasound probe (transducer) on a trajectory, receiving RF-echo signals from each probe position, and then transforming electrical energy into a light spot using grayscale on a monitor.[3,4]

US is a tomographic imaging technique. Sonograms (US images) are sections of certain thicknesses generated along the face of the transducer (contacts are with the tissue under examination) in the region of interest (**Fig. 1**). The depth of the section depends on the frequency of the transducer used. The sonogram is a composite of different shades of gray, the brightness of which depends on the frequency of the reflected echoes, which in turn depend on the ability of a tissue or structure to reflect or absorb sounds; this is known as echogenicity. With diagnostic US, tissues are classified based on their echogenicity in broad categories:

- Hyperechoic or echogenic, highly reflective tissues (very bright), such as osseous structures or cartilage
- Moderately echogenic (fairly bright), such as glands
- Hypoechoic (fairly dark), such as blood vessels and muscles
- Anechoic (very dark), such as fluids and air.

The collected echoes are processed very quickly by the US machine and images are almost instantly generated; this gives the impression of real-time imaging.

Diagnostic US has been used extensively for the assessment of soft tissue pathologic conditions of the head and neck with high-frequency transducers, including salivary gland disease (**Fig. 2**), neck vascular pathologic conditions, and nodal disease, as well as disease of floor of the mouth (**Fig. 3**). Guided fine-needle aspiration, measurement of tongue cancer thickness, and detection of metastasis to cervical lymph nodes are a few of the applications of US in soft tissue lesions.[3] In a recent study of 45 subjects, the diagnostic accuracy of US was 92.3% in cystic lesions, 87.5% in benign tumors, 81.8% in malignant tumors, 90% in space infections and abscesses, and 100% in lymphadenopathies (**Fig. 4**).[1]

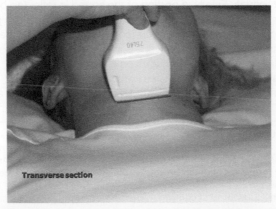

Transverse section

Fig. 1. The orientation of the transducer as it is applied on the body surface to be examined determines the section generated. In this case, a transverse section is produced along the red line.

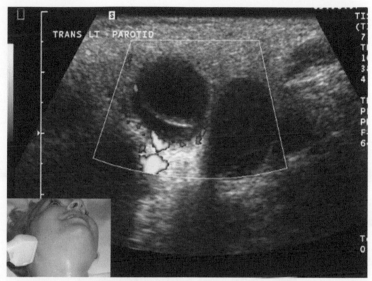

Fig. 2. Transverse section of the parotid salivary gland (Doppler US) illustrating the parotid gland, fairly echogenic (bright) and 2 large almost cystic, hypoechoic areas that show some internal debris. Note the high vascularity (hyperemia) depicted in the border of the hypoechoic areas, indicating inflammation. This was an abscess in the parotid gland.

The first introduction and application of US in dentistry was reported in 1953 by Lefkowitz.[5] In 1963, Baum and colleagues[6] used a 15-MHz transducer to display interior structures of teeth. However, the quality and clarity of the resulting RF signal was not satisfactory. Since then, US has been used to identify caries lesions, tooth fractures or cracks, soft tissue lesions, periodontal bony defects, maxillofacial fractures, and temporomandibular disorders, and to measure muscle and soft tissue thickness. The role of US in dental imaging and implant dentistry has been investigated.[3]

The acoustic characteristics of enamel, dentin, and soft tissue have been established but the acoustic characteristics of periodontal tissue have not yet been reported.[3,7] US has the ability to penetrate into most solids, including enamel and dentin, and to display caries and cracks that can hardly be seen in conventional radiography.[7] Enamel thickness can be measured with results satisfactorily close to the real enamel thickness using high-frequency transducer (ie, 25 MHz, 35 MHz).[8,9] In a study, a fractional Fourier transform with a 15-MHz transducer was used to measure enamel thickness and found to be a useful diagnostic tool to evaluate enamel thickness, tooth cracks, and possible restoration errors.[8] In a recent study, tooth, periodontal structures, dental implants, and mucocele could be displayed and measured using B-mode US with a 25-MHz high-frequency transducer produced for intraoral examination.[9]

According to a literature review assessing the feasibility of different diagnostic techniques for caries detection, there is still limited proof supporting each modality, mostly due to lack of standardization and limited clinical studies.[3] However, promising results have been reported regarding the capability of US to show caries lesions.[10]

US with high-frequency transducers can also be used to identify tooth fractures and cracks based on the similar principle used to assess enamel thickness and caries lesions.[3] Cracks at the dentinoenamel junction were identified in gold, amalgam, and porcelain restorations in a tooth phantom with a 19-MHz transducer. In extracted natural teeth, cracks could be displayed under porcelain and amalgam, and within a

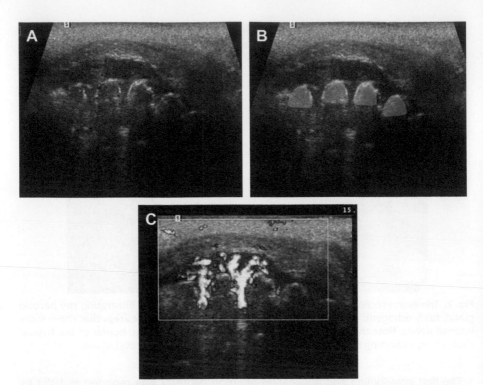

Fig. 3. Transverse section of the gingivae of the anterior maxilla. (*A*) The transducer was extraorally placed in contact with the upper lip, depicting a crescent-shaped, hypoechoic mass that expands between the anterior maxillary teeth. (*B*) Same section shaded to mark the mass under investigation (*red*) and the teeth (*blue*). (*C*) Doppler US of the same section depicting high vascularity of the mass; this mass was a pyogenic granuloma.

human molar, but not under gold. This may result from high acoustic impedance of gold restoration that transmits minimal acoustic energy.[11]

US can also give substantial diagnostic information about identification of periapical lesions, especially in the anterior region where the buccal bone is thin (**Fig. 5**). There

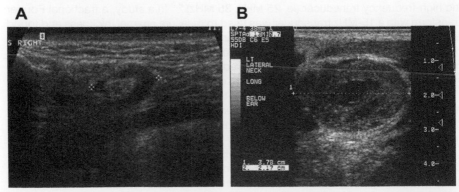

Fig. 4. (*A*) Normal (healthy) versus (*B*) abnormal (metastatic) cervical lymph nodes. Note the marked heterogeneity and the size of the metastatic lymph node, as well as central necrosis.

A

B

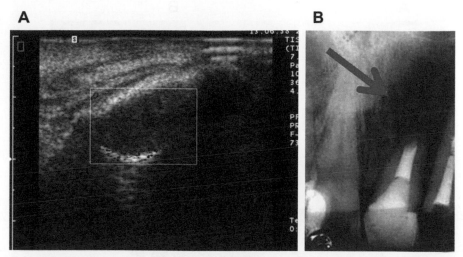

Fig. 5. (A) Sonogram of the periapical radiolucent lesion (*arrow*) around tooth #9 shown in (B) that presents an echogenic content and internal vascularization at the color Doppler US. (*Adapted from* Cotti E, Simbola V, Dettori C, et al. Echographic evaluation of bone lesions of endodontic origin: report of two cases in the same patient. J Endod 2006;32(9):902–3; with permission.)

has been an endless debate about diagnosis of periapical granuloma and cyst by conventional radiography; however, US seems to overcome this controversy.[2,12] The follow-up of postoperative healing of periapical lesions seems to be possible with US as well (**Fig. 6**).[12] This is a promising result for the trend toward radiation-free endodontics.

Displaying of periodontal ligament using US remains difficult because of complex anatomy and small impedance mismatch.[3] Recently, the feasibility of a custom-designed high-frequency (30–60 MHz) US to reconstruct high-resolution

A

B

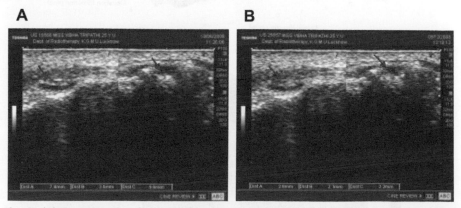

Fig. 6. (A) Postoperative (at 1 week) ultrasound image of a healing periapical lesion (*arrows*). (B) Postoperative (at 6 months) ultrasound image of a periapical lesion shows healing and bone formation (*arrows*). (*From* Tikku AP, Kumar S, Loomba K, et al. Use of ultrasound, color Doppler imaging and radiography to monitor periapical healing after endodontic surgery. J Oral Sci 2010;52(3):413; with permission.)

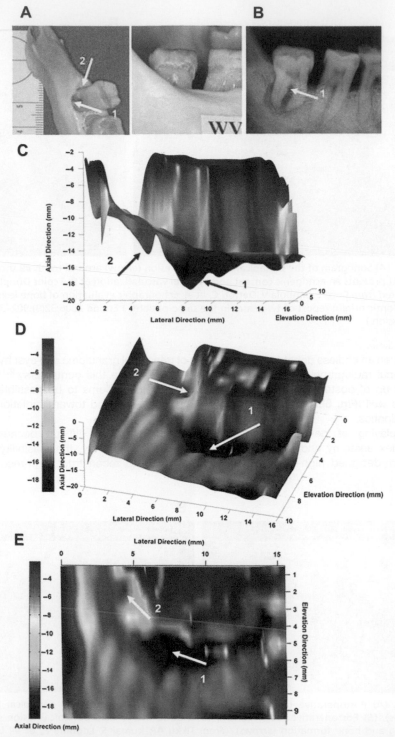

Fig. 7. Defective dentate dried cadaver mandible. (*A*) Two images of the mandible with showing 2 landmarks (*arrows*) around the third molar. (*B*) The corresponding X-ray

3-dimensional (3D) images of periodontal defects in human was investigated. It enabled reconstruction of 3D images of the bony defect in less than 30 seconds. US was shown to be a potential tool for the early diagnosis of severe forms of periodontal disease (**Fig. 7**).[13] However, more study is needed to confirm the use of US in showing bony defects and to establish a standard for clinical application.

Because acoustic characteristics of gingiva have not yet been established, results of studies performed with the aim of manufacturing an optimal ultrasonic device that can show oral mucosa thickness are not satisfactory.[3] On the other hand, determination of soft tissue thickness has clinical importance for the ability to identify different structures of the oral cavity and to make treatment plans in fields such as orthodontics (ie, proper orthodontic miniscrew selection)[14] and implant dentistry (ie, implant placement without incision and flap elevation).[15] US, using A-mode, has been found to be a potential aid to measure gingival thickness, especially with certain tooth types or the presence of thin gingiva.[14,16]

Implant surgery without incision and flap elevation requires precise determination of soft tissue thickness. During the subsequent healing period, location of implants can be challenging, especially if the implants are deeply submerged after thick connective tissue grafts.[3,17] Studies investigating the role of US in implant dentistry showed that US can locate submerged implants for surgical exposure following prosthodontic restoration.[15] Moreover, a new US device was introduced and found to be effective for the measurement of angular alignment between osteotome and the mandibular canal, and/or the floor of the maxillary sinus, during implant surgery.[18]

Maxillofacial fractures, muscle thickness, temporomandibular disorders, cysts, tumors, and vascular lesions have been displayed with US as well.[3]

US can be improved with a Doppler system (color Doppler or power Doppler) on a B-mode image. Color Doppler shows the mean velocity of moving tissues at a given time on a color scale, with red describing the flow toward the transducer and blue describing the flow away from the transducer. Power Doppler is a measure of the number of moving cells in a sample volume and is very sensitive for the blood flow in small vessels.[4,19] US, along with the color Doppler, enables display of the content and vascularization of lesions. Soft tissue lesions (ie, tongue cancer thickness, lymph node metastasis),[1] intraosseous lesions (ie, cysts, tumors),[20] pulpal blood flow,[21] and periapical lesions of endodontic origin,[12] are a few examples of what can be assessed with Doppler systems.

Unfortunately, the use of US in dentistry is still in its infancy; however, studies are very promising. Well-known features of US are that it is nonionizing, noninvasive, fast, cost-effective, painless, and reproducible; it provides real-time and simultaneous imaging of both hard and soft tissue; and it is easily tolerated by patients. One of the most striking feature is, because it is nonionizing, US can be performed as often as needed in a very short time. This is especially significant if planning or performing a surgery. However, dental applications for US are still not well-known by many practitioners, which may be a disadvantage to both practitioner and patient. Further studies should explore the capability of US, with the goal of making US a common tool in dentistry.

---

radiographic describing landmark #1 (*arrow*). (*C–E*) Different views of the 3D ultrasound jawbone surface image, which were able to detect different bony defects that could not be defined using X-ray images at landmark #1 (sever defect) and landmark #2 (early stage defect) (*arrows*). (*From* Mahmoud AM, Ngan P, Crout R, et al. High-resolution 3D ultrasound jawbone surface imaging for diagnosis of periodontal bony defects: an in vitro study. Ann Biomed Eng 2010;38(11):3419; with permission.)

REFERENCES

1. Pallagatti S, Sheikh S, Puri N, et al. To evaluate the efficacy of ultrasonography compared to clinical diagnosis, radiography and histopathological findings in the diagnosis of maxillofacial swellings. Eur J Radiol 2012;81(8): 1821–7.

2. Sandhu SS, Singh S, Arora S, et al. Comparative evaluation of advanced and conventional diagnostic AIDS for endodontic management of periapical lesions, an in vivo study. J Clin Diagn Res 2015;9(1):ZC01–4.

3. Marotti J, Heger S, Tinschert J, et al. Recent advances of ultrasound imaging in dentistry–a review of the literature. Oral Surg Oral Med Oral Pathol Oral Radiol 2013;115(6):819–32.

4. Musu D, Rossi-Fedele G, Campisi G, et al. Ultrasonography in the diagnosis of bone lesions of the jaws: a systematic review. Oral Surg Oral Med Oral Pathol Oral Radiol 2016;122(1):e19–29.

5. Lefkowitz W. Ultrasonics in dentistry. J Am Dent Assoc 1956;52(4):406–9.

6. Baum G, Greenwood I, Slawski S, et al. Observation of internal structures of teeth by ultrasonography. Science 1963;139(3554):495–6.

7. Culjat MO, Goldenberg D, Tewari P, et al. A review of tissue substitutes for ultrasound imaging. Ultrasound Med Biol 2010;36(6):861–73.

8. Harput S, Evans T, Bubb N, et al. Diagnostic ultrasound tooth imaging using fractional Fourier transform. IEEE Trans Ultrason Ferroelectr Freq Control 2011; 58(10):2096–106.

9. Salmon B, Le Denmat D. Intraoral ultrasonography: development of a specific high-frequency probe and clinical pilot study. Clin Oral Investig 2012;16(2): 643–9.

10. Hughes DA, Girkin JM, Poland S, et al. Investigation of dental samples using a 35MHz focused ultrasound piezocomposite transducer. Ultrasonics 2009;49(2): 212–8.

11. Singh RS, Culjat MO, Cho JC, et al. Penetration of radiopaque dental restorative materials using a novel ultrasound imaging system. Am J Dent 2007;20(4):221–6.

12. Tikku AP, Kumar S, Loomba K, et al. Use of ultrasound, color Doppler imaging and radiography to monitor periapical healing after endodontic surgery. J Oral Sci 2010;52(3):411–6.

13. Mahmoud AM, Ngan P, Crout R, et al. High-resolution 3D ultrasound jawbone surface imaging for diagnosis of periodontal bony defects: an in vitro study. Ann Biomed Eng 2010;38(11):3409–22.

14. Parmar R, Reddy V, Reddy SK, et al. Determination of soft tissue thickness at orthodontic miniscrew placement sites using ultrasonography for customizing screw selection. Am J Orthod Dentofacial Orthop 2016;150(4):651–8.

15. Culjat MO, Choi M, Singh RS, et al. Ultrasound detection of submerged dental implants through soft tissue in a porcine model. J Prosthet Dent 2008;99(3): 218–24.

16. Muller HP, Barrieshi-Nusair KM, Kononen E. Repeatability of ultrasonic determination of gingival thickness. Clin Oral Investig 2007;11(4):439–42.

17. Shah N, Bansal N, Logani A. Recent advances in imaging technologies in dentistry. World J Radiol 2014;6(10):794–807.

18. Machtei EE, Zigdon H, Levin L, et al. Novel ultrasonic device to measure the distance from the bottom of the osteotome to various anatomic landmarks. J Periodontol 2010;81(7):1051–5.

19. Anderson T, McDicken WN. The difference between colour Doppler velocity imaging and power Doppler imaging. Eur J Echocardiogr 2002;3(3):240–4.

20. Sumer AP, Danaci M, Ozen Sandikci E, et al. Ultrasonography and Doppler ultrasonography in the evaluation of intraosseous lesions of the jaws. Dentomaxillofac Radiol 2009;38(1):23–7.

21. Yoon MJ, Kim E, Lee SJ, et al. Pulpal blood flow measurement with ultrasound Doppler imaging. J Endod 2010;36(3):419–22.

Nuclear Medicine Imaging in the Dentomaxillofacial Region

Heidi R. Wassef, MD[a],*, Patrick M. Colletti, MD[b]

KEYWORDS

- Dentomaxillofacial • Nuclear medicine • ^{99m}Tc-MDP
- ^{18}F sodium fluoride bone scan • ^{18}F-FDG • Osteomyelitis • Condylar hyperplasia
- Temporomandibular disorder

KEY POINTS

- Nuclear medicine studies evaluate the physiology on a molecular level providing earlier detection of lesions before morphologic change is evident.
- ^{99m}Tc-MDP and ^{18}F-NaF PET bone scans aid in the detection of osseous tumor, infection, condylar hyperplasia, temporomandibular disorder and osteoradionecrosis and can assess bone graft viability.
- ^{99m}Tc-MDP and ^{18}F NaF PET bone scans detect osteomyelitis earlier than CT and 18F-FDG PET/CT can assess osteomyelitis complicated by fracture or surgery.
- ^{18}F-NaF PET/CT bone scan is more sensitive and specific than ^{99m}Tc-MDP for evaluation of osseous lesions.
- 18F-FDG PET/CT provides more accurate staging, restaging, response to treatment, and prognostic data for malignant disease than CT alone resulting in more precise patient management and improved outcomes.

NUCLEAR MEDICINE

Nuclear medicine displays physiologic processes at the molecular level. It is an imaging subspecialty that uses small amounts of radioactive material to diagnose and treat disease. Most radiopharmaceuticals administered are composed of a radioactive component (radioactive atom) bound to a physiologically active component. The choice of physiologically active component depends on the purpose of the scan. For example, if imaging of the bone is desired, technetium (^{99m}Tc) is bound to the bone-seeking agent, methylene diphosphonate (MDP),

Disclosure Statement: The authors have nothing to disclose.
[a] Department of Radiology, Keck School of Medicine of USC, PET Center, 1500 San Pablo Street, Los Angeles, CA 90033, USA; [b] Department of Radiology, Keck School of Medicine of USC, GNH 3549, Off Campus, Los Angeles, CA 90089-9311, USA
* Corresponding author. 1510 San Pablo Street, Los Angeles, CA 90033.
E-mail address: wassef@med.usc.edu

yielding ^{99m}Tc-MDP. Photons emitted by the ^{99m}Tc component are detected by scintillation crystals in the gamma camera. When the gamma camera rotates around the patient, three-dimensional single-photon emission computed tomography (SPECT) images are obtained, which have the advantage of improved image contrast and localization of lesions compared with planar scintigraphy. SPECT/computed tomography (CT) cameras also have the advantages of CT attenuation correction and anatomic correlation, which results in improved accuracy and diagnostic confidence.

Radiopharmaceuticals used with PET cameras emit positrons that undergo annihilation with electrons with emission of two 511-keV photons at 180°. These photons are detected by coincidence imaging when they strike the scintillation crystals. Coregistered CT data not only provide attenuation correction of the PET data but also excellent spatial resolution, helping to improve localization and characterization of lesions identified by PET. PET evaluates abnormalities on the molecular level before morphologic changes are evident on CT.[1]

BONE SCAN

Bone scans are sensitive studies of the entire skeleton. They are dependent on blood flow and adsorption on crystalline structure of hydroxyapatite. The inorganic mineral hydroxyapatite is made of calcium, phosphate, and hydroxyl ions. The most commonly used radiopharmaceutical for skeletal scintigraphy is ^{99m}Tc-MDP, which passively diffuses from the capillaries to the extravascular space. Because areas of increased tracer uptake correlate with areas of hyperemia and increased bone uptake, bone scans are well suited to evaluate osseous metastatic disease, osteomyelitis, temporomandibular joint (TMJ) disorder (TMD), inflammatory and degenerative arthritis, osteonecrosis of the mandible, condylar hyperplasia (CH), bone graft viability, and Paget disease. The anatomic changes related to these disorders are seen on radiography, whereas the activity is assessed by bone scintigraphy. A 10% increase in osteolytic or osteogenic activity is seen using nuclear imaging compared with the 40% to 50% decalcification needed to occur before changes are identified using conventional radiography.[2] Bone scans detect osseous lesions earlier and reveal more lesions than radiography. With renal excretion, high target to background ratio is reached at 2 to 3 hours. The patient is encouraged to be well hydrated to decrease the radiation dose to the bladder.[3] Images of areas of interest are obtained at 3 hours following the intravenous administration of 10 to 20 mCi of the radiopharmaceutical. Voiding before imaging is necessary because accumulation of excreted radiopharmaceutical in the bladder can obscure the pelvis. When osteomyelitis or cellulitis is suspected, radionuclide angiography followed by blood pool images are also obtained. Blood pool images in adults are obtained 5 minutes postinjection but in pediatrics are obtained immediately and no later than 4 minutes after flow because children have rapid bone metabolism.[4] Dual-head cameras can acquire anterior and posterior whole-body images simultaneously. It is important to avoid patient motion. Imaging may take 20 to 30 minutes or more. Higher resolution images are obtained with magnification views. To investigate smaller areas of interest, pinhole collimation improves spatial resolution but acquisition time is prolonged.[5]

^{18}F-FLUORIDE BONE SCAN

^{18}F-Fluoride is a highly sensitive bone-seeking PET tracer. ^{18}F-fluoride is produced in a cyclotron from ^{18}O-water. The most frequent indication for ^{18}F-fluoride PET is to evaluate suspected osseous metastatic disease but it can also aid in the diagnosis of osteomyelitis, TMD, inflammatory and degenerative arthritis, benign and malignant osseous lesions, osteonecrosis of the mandible, CH, bone graft viability, and Paget disease.[6] The uptake mechanism is similar to ^{99m}Tc-MDP reflecting blood flow and bone remodeling. ^{18}F-ions pass from plasma through the extravascular fluid space into the crystal.[6] The ^{18}F-ions chemisorb to the hydroxyapatite. Because ^{18}F-NaF is an analogue for the hydroxyl ion, it exchanges quickly for the hydroxyl ion on the surface of the hydroxyapatite matrix.[7] ^{18}F-Fluoride has the advantage of greater bone uptake compared with ^{99m}Tc-MDP and faster blood pool clearance. The first pass extraction is 70% to 100% for ^{18}F-fluoride as compared with 40% to 60% for ^{99m}Tc-MDP. Faster blood pool clearance is due to negligible protein binding. Good hydration helps speed excretion through the kidneys thus decreasing radiation dose and improving image quality. It rapidly clears the blood pool with only 10% remaining at 1 hour allowing earlier imaging compared with ^{99m}Tc-MDP. Other advantages include attenuation correction by CT and the ability to correlate the bone morphology in areas of increased ^{18}F-NaF uptake, yielding improved specificity.[5] ^{18}F-NaF has higher accuracy than ^{99m}Tc-MDP planar and SPECT bone scans.[7] The recommended dose is 185 to 370 MBq (5–10 mCi) for adults. The half-life of ^{18}F is 109 minutes. Imaging starts 45 to 60 minutes after tracer injection with 2- to 5-minute acquisitions per bed position.[7] For evaluation of metastatic disease, the entire skeleton is imaged.

^{18}F-FLUORODEOXYGLUCOSE PET

^{18}F-Fluorodeoxyglucose (^{18}F-FDG) is a PET radiopharmaceutical that is a glucose analogue. Areas of hypermetabolism have increased FDG uptake. ^{18}F-FDG PET shows abnormalities on the molecular level often before CT and MRI can detect abnormalities based on morphologic criteria. Neoplasm, infection, and inflammation are characterized by increased glucose use. ^{18}F-FDG PET is important in staging, restaging, and evaluating response to therapy in oncologic patients. Compared with CT and MRI, FDG PET is less limited by metallic artifacts. Patients are instructed to fast 4 to 6 hours to prevent insulin secretion, which would drive most of the injected dose to skeletal muscle and myocardium and decrease FDG uptake by tumors. Blood glucose is checked before FDG injection where ideal levels should be less than 150 to 200 mg/dL. The patient is instructed to avoid strenuous exercise during the 24 hours before the study to prevent excessive FDG uptake by the muscles. A total of 10 mCi of FDG is injected and imaging starts 45 to 60 minutes following injection. For most malignancies except melanoma and primary osseous neoplasms, imaging is from the level of the skull base to the midthighs. CT imaging is fast (60–70 seconds), whereas the PET component takes 30 to 45 minutes. CT resolution is 0.3 mm and PET resolution is 4 to 6 mm. The PET and CT images are fused after imaging the patient in the same position. The CT data are used for attenuation correction of the PET data. The standardized uptake value is a semiquantitative measure of the amount of hypermetabolism.[1] **Table 1** lists effective doses of various diagnostic radiologic studies.

INFECTION

CT and MRI are sensitive in evaluating location and extent of soft tissue infection and possible complications including abscess formation, osteomyelitis, airway narrowing, and vascular compromise. Triple-phase ^{99m}Tc bone scanning can diagnose

Table 1
Effective doses of dentomaxillofacial imaging examinations[8,9]

Examination	Effective Dose (mSv)
Intraoral radiography	0.005
Panoramic radiography	0.01
Dental cone beam CT	0.177
Posteroanterior and lateral chest radiography	0.1
Head CT	2
Chest CT	7
Abdomen CT	8
Whole-body ^{99m}Tc-MDP (25 mCi)	6.3
Whole-body ^{18}F-fluoride PET (10 mCi)	8.9
Whole-body ^{18}F-FDG PET (10 mCi)	14.1
Yearly radiation dose from background sources of radiation in the United States	3.1

osteomyelitis earlier than CT. If there is hardware at the site of suspected osteomyelitis a white blood cell scan and sulfur colloid scans or FDG PET are preferred. ^{18}F-FDG PET is superior to MDP bone scan for distinguishing soft tissue and bone infections and diagnosing osteomyelitis complicated by fracture or surgery. FDG uptake is increased at sites of fracture for approximately 1 month and following surgery for 6 months.[10] Increased osseous FDG uptake after 6 months is likely caused by osteomyelitis. Bone scans and FDG PET are not limited by hardware artifacts like CT and MRI.

Garré sclerosing osteomyelitis is a chronic nonsuppurative osteomyelitis most frequently affecting the mandible and associated with odontogenic infections. It mainly affects children and young adults. The classic radiographic appearance is "onion skin," representing several layers of periosteal proliferation of the cortex (**Fig. 1**).[11]

INFLAMMATORY DISEASE

Periodontal disease can be coincidentally detected on ^{99m}Tc-MDP and ^{18}F-fluoride PET bone scans in patients being evaluated for osseous metastases and on ^{18}F-FDG PET in patients being evaluated for head and neck malignancy (**Fig. 2**).

SJÖGREN SYNDROME

Sjögren syndrome (SS) is an autoimmune disease that is 10 times more common in women than men and is usually diagnosed between the age of 45 and 55. It can develop as a complication of other autoimmune diseases, such as rheumatoid arthritis or lupus. Lymphocytic infiltration of exocrine organs causes the patient to present with sicca symptoms, such as xerophthalmia (dry eyes), xerostomia (dry mouth), and parotid enlargement. Loss of salivary gland function leads to xerostomia. Salivary gland biopsy, sialography, MRI sialography, ultrasound, or Raman spectroscopy can evaluate the salivary glands or saliva.

Salivary scintigraphy provides information on the gland function. After the intravenous injection of 5 mCi of ^{99}Tc-sodium pertechnetate, it is taken up by the gland within 10 minutes and secreted into mouth by 20 to 30 minutes. In SS, pertechnetate concentration in the gland and secretion into mouth is decreased.[12]

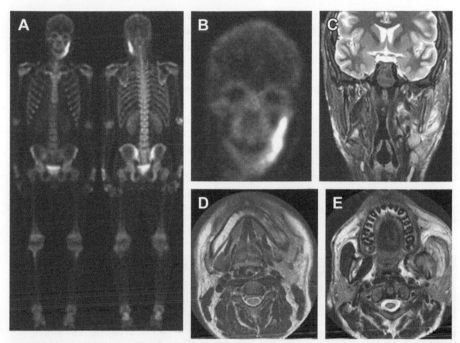

Fig. 1. Garré sclerosing osteomyelitis. An 18-year-old man with intense ^{99m}Tc-MDP uptake in the left mandible seen on anterior and posterior whole-body images (A) and anterior image of the head (B) consistent with osteomyelitis. He had a history of multiple dental procedures. Coronal STIR (C) and axial T2 (D, E) images reveal low signal intensity in the left maxilla with extension of the infection to the adjacent soft tissues.

^{99}Tc pertechnetate salivary gland scintigraphy can differentiate between chronic obstructive parotitis and SS. In the former, uptake is normal and excretion is decreased, and in SS uptake and excretion are diminished.[13] In a study of 111 patients with suspected SS, percentage uptake was the quantitative parameter with the highest diagnostic accuracy.[14]

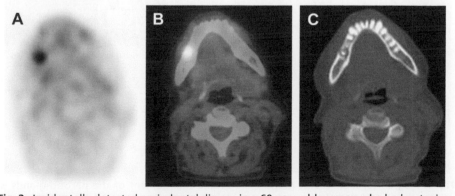

Fig. 2. Incidentally detected periodontal disease in a 60-year-old woman who had restaging FDG PET/CT for colon cancer. Focal hypermetabolism on FDG PET (A) and fused PET/CT (B) and widening of the periodontal ligament spaces in the second right molar on CT (C) are consistent with periodontal disease.

When MRI sialography and salivary scintigraphy were compared in the diagnosis of SS, MRI sialography had higher specificity and positive predictive value and salivary scintigraphy showed higher sensitivity. Overall diagnostic accuracy for MRI sialography was 83% and for scintigraphy was 72%.[15] A meta-analysis of six studies that included 488 patients and 447 control subjects from Europe and Asia showed that diagnostic accuracy of sialography is comparable with salivary ultrasound in patients with SS.[16]

A study of 213 patients with suspected SS evaluated multiple quantitative salivary scintigraphy parameters. They found that a new scoring system that combined pertechnetate ejection fraction following vitamin C stimulation with serology, ocular examination, and minor salivary gland biopsy yielded specificity similar to the 2002 American-European Consensus Group and 2012 American College of Rheumatology criteria, but improved the sensitivity significantly.[17,18] The inflammatory component of SS is well seen on PET/CT with intense FDG uptake in the affected glands (**Fig. 3**).

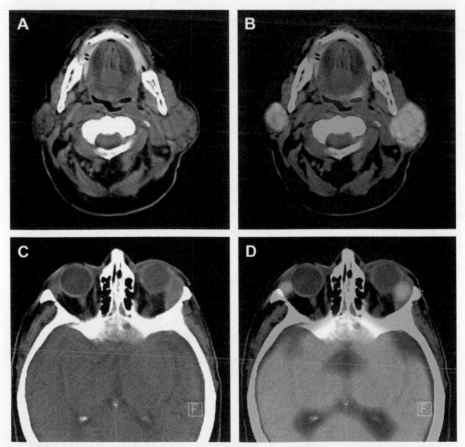

Fig. 3. Sjögren syndrome. Left greater than right enlargement of the parotid glands is seen on axial CT (*A*) and bilateral parotid hypermetabolism on axial fused PET/CT (*B*). Similarly, left greater than right lacrimal gland enlargement is seen on axial CT (*C*) with bilateral hypermetabolism on fused PET/CT (*D*) in a patient with active Sjögren syndrome.

SAPHO SYNDROME

The SAPHO (synovitis, acne, pustulosis, hyperostosis, osteitis) syndrome is rare. It occurs in patients between the ages of 30 and 50 years. Arthritis occurs most commonly (65%–90%) at the sternocostoclavicular region and least commonly (11%) in the TMJ. Bilateral sternoclavicular uptake is typical of but not sensitive for the diagnosis. Bone scintigraphy demonstrates sites of hyperostosis and osteitis, some of which may not be apparent on radiographs.[18]18F-FDG PET also detects areas of synovitis.

TEMPOROMANDIBULAR JOINT DISORDER

99mTc-MDP SPECT/CT allows correlation of increased MDP bone uptake with morphologic changes on CT in the TMJ. 99mTc-MDP SPECT/CT imaging has a sensitivity, specificity, and accuracy of 100%, 90.91%, and 96.97%, respectively, for correlation with signs and symptoms of TMD.[2] The overall accuracy is higher than SPECT alone. SPECT imaging can also monitor effect of therapy. Six-month splint therapy resulted in a lower bone uptake ratio of affected versus nonaffected TMJ and affected TMJ versus occipital bone uptake and this correlated with improvement in TMJ pain.[19]

A study of 48 TMJs in 24 patients found that the TMJ-to-skull ^{18}F-PET bone uptake ratio had higher sensitivity and accuracy compared with 9mTc-MDP bone ratio in diagnosing temporomandibular disease with osteoarthritis and differentiating it from TMD with anterior disk displacement (**Fig. 4**).[20]

ASSESSMENT OF CONDYLAR HYPERPLASIA

Condylar hyperplasia (CH) is excessive and asymmetric growth of a mandibular condyle. Although painless, CH causes asymmetric facial deformities, mandibular deviation, malocclusion, and articular dysfunction.[21] CT evaluates the condylar morphology and bony changes over time. The bone scan determines if there is active growth and remodeling. Combined SPECT/CT can evaluate the morphology and the activity aiding in diagnosis and patient management. A bone scan with greater than 10% uptake in one condyle compared with the contralateral condyle establishes CH by demonstrating unilateral growth (**Fig. 5**). The quantitative assessment done by evaluating the counts in regions of interest in both condyles helps determine the treatment course. The presence of coexistent unilateral or asymmetric osteoarthritis can limit the quantitative assessment.[22] SPECT has a higher sensitivity than planar imaging with similar specificity.[23] In a comparison of planar bone scan, SPECT, and SPECT/CT, both SPECT and SPECT/CT had a sensitivity of 80%. Diagnostic accuracy for planar bone scan is only 47.6%. Diagnostic accuracy, sensitivity, and specificity for SPECT/CT are 85.8%, 80%, and 100%, respectively.[24] Intense uptake on SPECT bone scan was also found to correlate with larger and more frequent islands of cartilage in the surgical specimen following surgery.[25] A study evaluating the role of ^{18}F-fluoride PET/CT in the diagnosis of CH found that the mean standardized uptake value max of the affected side was 9.18 and of the unaffected side was 6.2 and the percentage difference was 16.87%.[26] Laverick and colleagues[27] also found ^{18}F to correctly diagnose active CH. In conclusion, SPECT/CT and ^{18}F-fluoride PET/CT can help establish the diagnosis of CH and determine appropriate management.

PAGET DISEASE

Paget disease, also called osteitis deformans, is the second most common bone disease of the elderly following osteoporosis.[28] The increased bone turnover in Paget disease results in structurally disorganized remodeling and enlarged bone. Lumbar

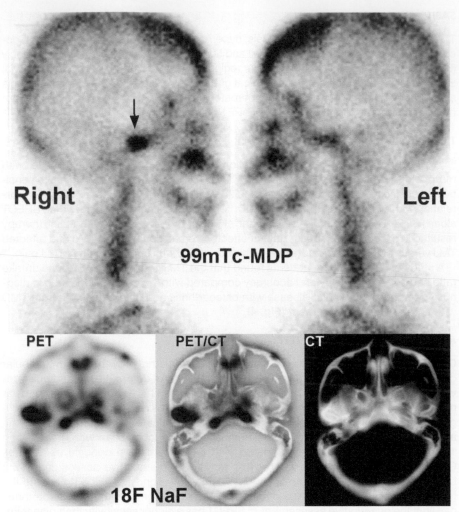

Fig. 4. Temporomandibular disease. 99mTc-MDP bone scan (*top images*) and 18F-NaF PET, PET/CT, and CT (*bottom images*) all demonstrate a deformed, sclerotic, hyperactive degenerated right temporomandibular joint (*arrow*). (*From* Lee JW, Lee SM, Kim S-J, et al. Clinical utility of fluoride-18 positron emission tomography/CT in temporomandibular disorder with osteoarthritis comparisons with 99mTc-MDP bone scan. Dentomaxillofac Radiol 2013;42:2; with permission.)

vertebra and skull are most frequently involved. The three major phases include (1) the lytic phase dominated by osteoclastic resorption; (2) the mixed phase, which includes osteoclastic and osteoblastic changes with predominant osteoblastic activity; and (3) the blastic phase characterized by decreasing osteoblastic activity. The diagnosis is usually made by radiography with typical findings including subperiosteal cortical thickening and coarsening of the trabecular pattern. Radiography may underestimate the extent of the disease because conversion of normal bone to pagetic bone is seen on scintigraphy before radiographic changes are evident. 99mTc-MDP and 18F-fluoride PET bone scans are sensitive examinations. Intense radionuclide uptake in the region of abnormal bone is seen in all three phases of Paget disease.[28] The complications of Paget disease, such as pathologic fractures, skeletal deformities, and arthropathy, are

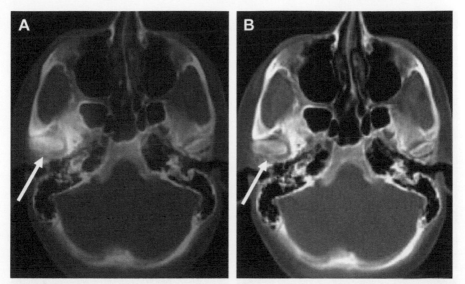

Fig. 5. Condylar hyperplasia. A 21-year-old woman with facial asymmetry was referred for assessment of condylar growth activity. SPECT/CT confirmed increased condylar MDP uptake (*A*) and low-dose CT showed enlarged condylar head consistent with the diagnosis of active condylar hyperplasia (*B*). (*From* Derlin T, Busch JD, Habermann CR. 99mTc-MDP SPECT/CT for assessment of condylar hyperplasia. Clin Nucl Med 2013;38(1):e49; with permission.)

better evaluated with CT and neurologic symptoms and malignant transformation is better evaluated with MRI.

MALIGNANT NEOPLASMS

Head and neck cancers account for 3% of all cancers in the United States and are the cause of death for 12,000 Americans per year.[29] Most head and neck cancers are squamous cell carcinomas arising from the mucosal lining of the upper aerodigestive tract (**Fig. 6**). PET/CT has a higher sensitivity and specificity for staging head and neck cancers that are squamous cell carcinomas compared with contrast-enhanced CT (CECT) or MRI (**Figs. 7** and **8**). After therapy, changes in tumor metabolism occur before morphologic changes. This allows FDG PET/CT to provide earlier and more accurate evaluation of response to treatment and restaging. It can distinguish between malignant and benign disease especially when surgery has greatly altered the anatomy (**Fig. 9**). PET data also provide important prognostic information for more individualized surveillance and therapy planning. Higher FDG uptake correlates with poorly differentiated tumors and worse prognosis. It is hoped that PET will soon be able to differentiate tumors that would and those that would not respond to radiation therapy (RT). Patients with the former can be treated with RT with or without chemotherapy and can be spared neck dissection. Patients who would not respond to RT can have early surgical resection and be spared the sequelae of RT. RT planning based on PET yields more accurate and often smaller radiation fields compared with that based on CECT (**Fig. 10**). PET has a high sensitivity in identifying recurrent, synchronous, and metachronous tumor. FDG-PET/CT can localize the primary tumor in 22% to 44% of patients with unknown primary head and neck cancer after standard work-up.[30]

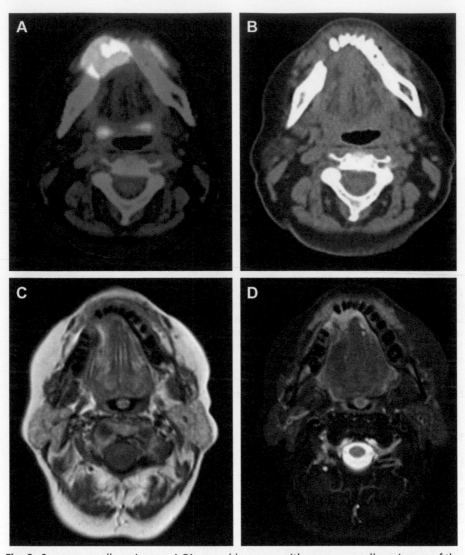

Fig. 6. Squamous cell carcinoma. A 51-year-old woman with squamous cell carcinoma of the right mandible involving the lip and oral cavity. Hypermetabolic tumor is seen on fused PET/CT (*A*) and osseous destruction is seen on CT (*B*). Tumor has low signal on T1 (*C*) and high signal on fat-suppressed T2-weighted axial MRI images (*D*).

Similarly, FDG PET/CT is more sensitive and specific in the evaluation of lymphoma, melanoma, and metastatic disease to the maxillofacial region compared with CECT (**Fig. 11**). Metastatic disease to the oral and maxillofacial region is rare. The most frequent primaries are breast cancer, renal cell cancer, prostate cancer, and melanoma in the United States and lung, thyroid, liver, esophagus, and stomach cancers in China.[31] This portends a poor prognosis. A study of 62 patients with oral and maxillofacial metastases found that all patients died within 5 years. The mean survival time was 1.09 ± 0.20 years for men and 1.40 ± 0.30 years for women.[32] Although not routinely used, puffed cheek

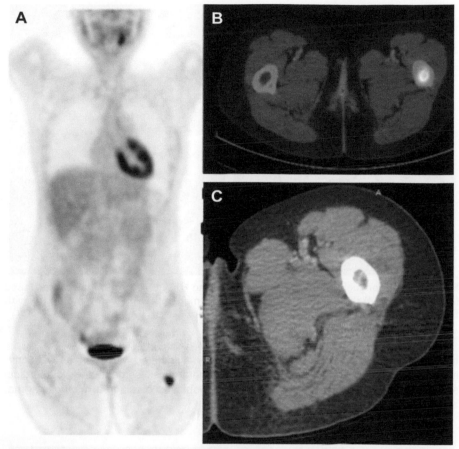

Fig. 7. Metastatic nasopharyngeal cancer to the femur. A 40-year-old woman with stage IV nasopharyngeal carcinoma treated with chemotherapy. Restaging FDG PET/CT revealed left femoral metastasis from nasopharyngeal carcinoma on whole-body maximum intensity projection PET (*A*) and axial fused PET/CT (*B*). The biopsy-proven metastasis was not clearly visible on axial CT (*C*).

technique improves localization and extent of oral and oropharyngeal lesions and decreases dental amalgam artifact.[33] FDG-PET/CT has become the primary imaging modality for staging, evaluating response to therapy, and restaging in head and neck primary, lymphoma, and selected metastatic neoplasms.

OSSEOUS NEOPLASTIC DISEASE

^{18}F-NaF PET has a higher sensitivity and specificity in detecting osseous metastases, compared with ^{99m}Tc-based bone scintigraphy. Although radiation dose is slightly higher than MDP, ^{18}F-NaF PET is faster and more convenient for patients. ^{18}F-NaF PET is superior to ^{18}F- FDG PET in osteoblastic bone tumors, whereas the latter is superior in osteolytic bone tumors. FDG PET has a higher sensitivity and diagnostic power compared with bone marrow biopsy for the detection of osseous involvement by Hodgkin disease.[34] Keratocystic odontogenic tumors that undergo malignant

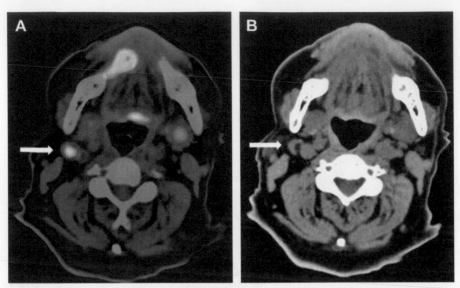

Fig. 8. Staging tongue cancer by FDG PET/CT. Staging FDG PET/CT for tongue cancer. Fused (*arrows*) PET/CT (*A*) shows hypermetabolism in a benign-appearing 1-cm lymph node with fatty hilum seen on CT (*B*) consistent with malignancy.

transformation into squamous cell carcinoma are associated with intense FDG activity. FDG PET/CT is used for the initial staging, therapy assessment, and postsurgical surveillance of malignant ameloblastoma, ameloblastic carcinoma, plasmacytoma, and multiple myeloma.[35]

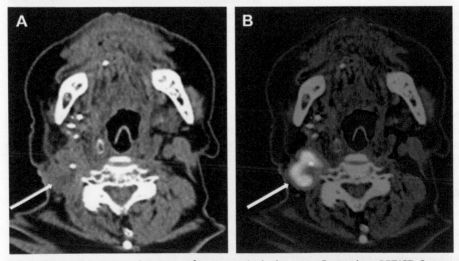

Fig. 9. Recurrent tumor in area of postsurgical changes. Restaging PET/CT 2 years following treatment shows on CT (*A*) postoperative changes status post partial right glossectomy and modified right neck dissection. Recurrent disease is well depicted on PET-CT (*B*) as level II conglomerate adenopathy (*arrows*).

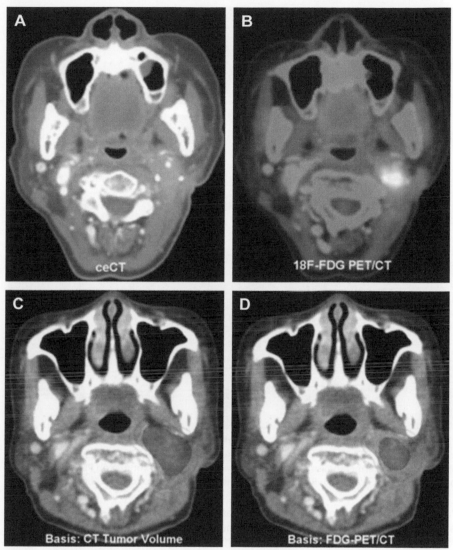

Fig. 10. PET/CT in radiation therapy planning. A 62-year-old man with recurrent nasopharyngeal squamous cell cancer. Soft tissue in the left carotid space is seen (*A*) on CECT. PET/CT (*B*) allows differentiation of recurrent tumor from post-treatment fibrosis, allowing accurate radiation planning. The smaller radiation field based on PET (*D*) compared with the area based on CECT (*C*) helps avoid radiation of at-risk structures in the neck and the associated sequelae. (*From* Wassef H, Hanna N, Colletti PM. PET/CT in head-neck malignancies. PET Clin 2016;11(3):223; with permission.)

EVALUATION OF BONE GRAFTS

Angiography assesses vascular patency only and the contrast may damage the endothelium of the intima at the anastomosis whereas bone scans have the unique feature of evaluating vascular patency and metabolic viability of the bone graft.[36,37] Bone scans are used to evaluate bone viability in different clinical scenarios, such as

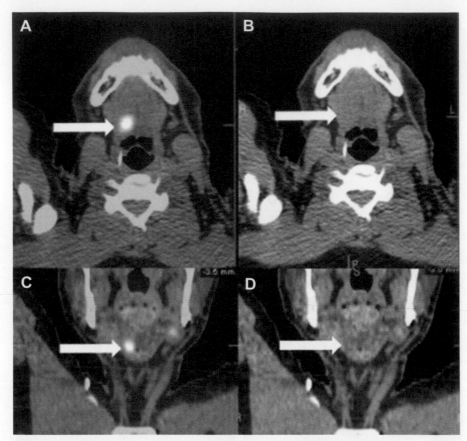

Fig. 11. Metastatic rectal cancer. A 73-year-old man with history of rectal carcinoma had a surveillance FDG PET/CT. Axial fused PET/CT (*A*), CT (*B*), coronal PET/CT (*C*), and CT (*D*) are shown. Focal hypermetabolism at the right paramedian base of tongue on PET was not visible on noncontrast CT (*arrows*). Biopsy revealed metastatic disease from rectal carcinoma.

"avascular necrosis, septic embolism, frostbite lesions and osteonecrosis, and to evaluate the results of surgical treatment in cases of avascular necrosis,"[4] 99mTc-MDP and 18F-fluoride have high affinity for hydroxyapatite crystals. Uptake of both tracers indicates bone viability by demonstrating vascular supply and osteoblast activity. Planar gamma camera images are obtained during the vascular phase with individual images of 1 second per frame for 60 seconds during 99mTc-labelled phosphonate injection. Blood pool images are obtained 5 minutes after injection. The delayed-phase images are obtained at 3 (2–4) hours. A pinhole collimator allows for higher resolution and magnification of the image with proper positioning and immobilization.

Furr and colleagues[38] retrospectively evaluated 205 fibular bone grafts in patients with partial mandibulectomy following head and neck cancer or trauma. Fifteen flaps clinically suspected to be threatened 4 to 153 days following surgery were evaluated with three-phase bone scans. They found that bone scans have high specificity. All grafts determined to be nonviable by the bone scans were proven so surgically. All grafts read as viable or potentially viable were viable. They used a four-point scale comparing the graft with normal mandibular and soft tissue uptake.

An evaluation of 60 bone scans with SPECT of 39 bone grafts in 36 patients in another study found that transplant to cranium ratio greater than one as early as 6 to 11 days after mandibular reconstruction with microvascularized bone grafts indicated success-ful surgery and transplant to cranium ratio less than one predicted necrosis.[39] A smaller study of 10 patients by Harada sought to understand the physiology of viable mandib-ular microvascularized bone grafts over time using three-phase bone scanning.[36] Sequential bone scanning was performed from 7 days to 12 months following surgery. Anastomotic patency was assessed by the flow phase. Blood pool activity decreased with time representing remodeling. Delayed bone images revealed peak activity at 1 week after surgery and started decreasing after 4 weeks. The advantage of osteosyn-thesis evaluation by ^{18}F-fluoride is the ability to quantify blood flow and fluoride influx in the areas between the graft bone and native bone.[40] ^{18}F-fluoride and ^{99m}Tc-MDP bone scans are accurate tools in the early evaluation of bone graft viability the surgeon with surgical and reconstructive management of bone grafts.

MEDICATION-RELATED OSTEONECROSIS OF THE JAW

Biphosphonates are used to treat osteoporosis; malignant bone disease, such as lytic breast metastases; multiple myeloma; and Paget disease. Biphosphonates inhibit osteoclastic activity.

Bisphosphonate-related osteonecrosis of the jaw (BRONJ) is a well-known complica-tion of bisphosphonate therapy. The name has changed to medication-related osteo-necrosis of the jaw (MRONJ) because antiangiogenic therapies have also been implicated. Three criteria are required to make the diagnosis of MRONJ according to the American Association of Maxillofacial Surgeons: (1) current or prior treatment with antiresorptive or antiangiogenic agents, (2) no history of local radiation therapy, and (3) persistently exposed bone in the maxillofacial region for more than 8 weeks.[41]

There is often a history of dental caries or recent dental procedures. MRONJ may be asymptomatic or painful. The necrotic area can progress to soft tissue infection, oste-omyelitis, or pathologic fracture. The predilection of the jaw to BRONJ may be due to the high turnover of bone and the exposure of the jaw to numerous sources of trauma, such as dental procedures, mastication, and infection, such as periodontal disease.[42] The estimated cumulative incidence of MRONJ in patients who had intravenous bisphosphonate is between 0.8% and 12% and between 0.01% and 0.06% for those who had oral biphosphonates.[43–45] The incidence of BRONJ is lower for patients being treated for osteoporosis than those treated for malignancy because phosphonates are given at higher doses and frequency in oncology patients.[46] Dental examination and treatment before the initiation of bisphosphonate therapy decreases the incidence of MRONJ.[43] MDP uptake has been found to correlate with MRONJ stage and may help with prognosis. ^{18}F-fluoride PET/CT is more sensitive and specific in the detec-tion of BRONJ compared with ^{99m}Tc bone scan because of the better spatial resolu-tion, correlation with CT findings, and the multiplanar image evaluation. ^{18}F-fluoride PET and contrast-enhanced MRI demonstrate more extensive histologically confirmed disease compared with panoramic views from cone beam CT and clinical examination.[44] ^{18}F-FDG can assess the severity of MRONJ and the response to treat-ment with decreasing uptake indicating good response (**Fig. 12**).[47]

OTHER SEQUELAE OF THERAPY FOR HEAD AND NECK CARCINOMA

FDG PET can detect other sequelae of treatment including parotitis; esophagitis; mucositis; aspiration pneumonia; infection; and secondary cancers by demonstrating hypermetabolism associated with inflammation, infection, and neoplasms.

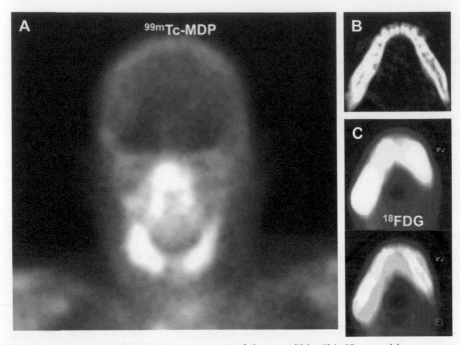

Fig. 12. Zoledronic acid–related osteonecrosis of the mandible. This 53-year-old woman was treated for stage 4 breast cancer with chemotherapy and zoledronic acid. ^{99m}Tc-MDP (*A*), CT (*B*), and FDG PET/CT (*C*) demonstrate mixed sclerotic and lytic bone with increased turnover and metabolism (max standardized uptake value = 8).

PHYSIOLOGIC AND MOLECULAR IMAGING

^{99m}Tc-MDP and ^{18}F-fluoride bone scans can detect osteomyelitis earlier than radiographs and CT and aid in the diagnosis of TMD. They can evaluate the activity of CH, extent of Paget disease, and viability of bone grafts. ^{18}F-FDG PET/CT can

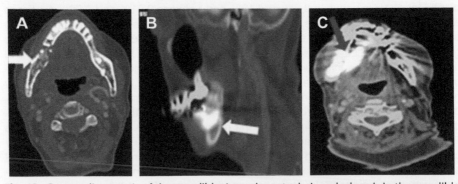

Fig. 13. Osteoradionecrosis of the mandible. Irregular osteolysis and sclerosis in the mandible on CT (*A, arrow*) is consistent with osteoradionecrosis 2 years after radiotherapy. Hypermetabolism is seen in the area of osteoradionecrosis on PET/CT (*B, arrow*). Biopsy-proven tongue carcinoma was discovered on surveillance PET/CT (*C, arrow*) 3 years after radiation. Surveillance PET/CT may detect second primaries in this patient population with high incidence of secondary head and neck, lung, and esophageal cancers. (*From* Wassef H, Hanna N, Colletti PM. PET/CT in head-neck malignancies. PET Clin 2016;11(3):228; with permission.)

distinguish between soft tissue and bone infections and diagnose osteomyelitis complicated by fracture or surgery. FDG PET is more accurate and has a major role in staging, restaging, and assessing response to therapy for head and neck malignancies and in detecting sequelae of therapy. It accurately determines the extent of osteoradionecrosis (**Fig. 13**). Physiologic and molecular imaging provided by nuclear medicine may have an increasing role in the management of diseases of the dentomaxillofacial region.

REFERENCES

1. Kapoor V, McCook BM, Torok FS. An introduction to PET-CT imaging. Radiographics 2004;24(2):523–43.
2. Coutinho A, Fenyo-Pereira M, Lauria L, et al. The role of SPECT/CT with 99mTc-MDP image fusion to diagnose temporomandibular dysfunction. Oral Surg Oral Med Oral Pathol Oral Radiol Endod 2006;101:224–30.
3. Mettler F, Guibertea M. Skeletal system. In: Essentials of nuclear medicine imaging. 6th edition. London: Elsevier Health Sciences; 2002. p. 273.
4. Roca I, Barber I, Fontecha CG, et al. Evaluation of bone viability. Pediatr Radiol 2013;43:393–405.
5. Segall G, Delbeke D, Stabin M, et al. SNM practice guideline for sodium 18F-fluoride PET/CT bone scan 1. 0. J Nucl Med 2010;51(11):1813–20.
6. Blau M, Ganatra R, Bender M. 18 F-fluoride for bone imaging. Semin Nucl Med 1972;2(1):31–7.
7. Czernin J, Satyamurthy N, Schiepers C. Molecular mechanisms of bone ^{18}F-NaF deposition. J Nucl Med 2010;51(12):1826–9.
8. Mettler FA, Huda W, Yoshizumi TT, et al. Effective doses in radiology and diagnostic nuclear medicine: a catalog. Radiology 2008;248(1):254–63.
9. Li G. Patient radiation dose and protection from cone-beam computed tomography. Imaging Sci Dent 2013;43(2):63–9.
10. Dioguardi P, Gaddam S, Zhuang H, et al. FDG PET assessment of osteomyelitis: a review. PET Clin 2012;7(2):161–79.
11. Suma R, Vinay C, Shashikanth M, et al. Garre's sclerosing osteomyelitis. J Indian Soc Pedod Prev Dent 2007;25(5):30–3.
12. Aoun G, Nasseh I, Berberi A. Evaluation of the oral component of Sjögren's syndrome: an overview. J Int Soc Prev Community Dent 2016;6(4):278–84.
13. Wu CB, Xi H, Zho Q, et al. The diagnostic value of technetium 99m pertechnetate salivary gland scintigraphy in patients with certain salivary gland diseases. J Oral Maxillofac Surg 2015;73(3):443–50.
14. Infante JR, García L, Rayo JI, et al. Diagnostic contribution of quantitative analysis of salivary scintigraphy in patients with suspected Sjögren's syndrome. Rev Esp Med Nucl Imagen Mol 2016;35(3):145–51.
15. Tonami H, Higashi K, Matoba M, et al. A comparative study between MR sialography and salivary gland scintigraphy in the diagnosis of Sjögren syndrome. J Comput Assist Tomogr 2001;25(2):262–8.
16. Song GG, Lee YH. Diagnostic accuracies of sialography and salivary ultrasonography in Sjögren's syndrome patients: a meta-analysis. Clin Exp Rheumatol 2014; 32(4):516–22.
17. Chen J, Zhao X, Liu H, et al. A point-scoring system for the clinical diagnosis of sjögren's syndrome based on quantified SPECT imaging of salivary gland. PLoS One 2016;11(5):e0155666.
18. Rukavina I. SAPHO syndrome: a review. J Child Orthop 2015;9(1):19–27.

19. Hersek N, Canay S, Caner B. Bone SPECT imaging of patients with internal derangement of temporomandibular joint before and after splint therapy. Surg Oral Med Oral Pathol Oral Radiol Endod 2002;94(5):576–80.
20. Lee JW, Lee SM, Kim SJ, et al. Clinical utility of fluoride-18 positron emission tomography/CT in temporomandibular disorder with osteoarthritis: comparisons with 99mTc-MDP bone scan. Dentomaxillofac Radiol 2013;42:2.
21. Portelli M, Gatto E, Matarese G, et al. Unilateral condylar hyperplasia: diagnosis, clinical aspects and operative treatment. A case report. Eur J Paediatr Dent 2015; 16(2):99–102.
22. Yang Z, Reed T, Longino BH. Bone scintigraphy SPECT/CT evaluation of mandibular condylar hyperplasia. J Nucl Med Technol 2016;44(1):49–51.
23. Saridin CP, Raijmakers PG, Tuinzing DB, et al. Bone scintigraphy as a diagnostic method in unilateral hyperactivity of the mandibular condyles: a review and meta-analysis of the literature. Int J Oral Maxillofac Surg 2011;40(1):11–7.
24. Agarwal KK, Mukherjee A, St A, et al. Incremental value of single-photon emission computed tomography/computed tomography in the diagnosis of active condylar hyperplasia. Nucl Med Commun 2017;38(1):29–34.
25. Martin-Granizo R, Garcia-Rielo JM, De la Sen O, et al. Correlation between single photon emission computed tomography and histopathologic findings in condylar hyperplasia of the temporomandibular joint. J Craniomaxillofac Surg 2017;45(6): 839–44.
26. Ahmed R, Singh SP, Mittal BR, et al. Role of fluorine-18 fluoride PET-CT scan in the assessment of unilateral condylar hyperplasia in faciomandibular asymmetry patients: a preliminary study. Nucl Med Commun 2016;37(3):263–72.
27. Laverick S, Bounds G, Wong WL. [18F]-fluoride positron emission tomography for imaging condylar hyperplasia. Br J Oral Maxillofac Surg 2009;47(3):196–9.
28. Theodorou DJ, Theodorou SJ, Kakitsubata Y. Imaging of Paget disease of bone and its musculoskeletal complications: review. Am J Roentgenol 2011;196(6): S64–75.
29. Siegel RL, Miller KD, Jemal A. Cancer statistics. CA Cancer J Clin 2015;2015(65): 5–29.
30. Karapolat I, Kumanlıoğlu K. Impact of FDG-PET/CT for the detection of unknown primary tumours in patients with cervical lymph node metastases. Mol Imaging Radionucl Ther 2012;21(2):63–8.
31. Shen ML, Kang J, Wen YL, et al. Metastatic tumors to the oral and maxillofacial region: a retrospective study of 19 cases in West China and review of the Chinese and English literature. J Oral Maxillofac Surg 2009;67(4):718–37.
32. Friedrich RE, Abadi M. Distant metastases and malignant cellular neoplasms encountered in the oral and maxillofacial region: analysis of 92 patients treated at a single institution. Anticancer Res 2010;30(5):1843–8.
33. Chang CY, Yang BH, Lin KH, et al. Feasibility and incremental benefit of puffed-cheek 18F-FDG PET/CT on oral cancer patients. Clin Nucl Med 2013;38(10): e374–8.
34. Cheng G, Alavi A. Value of 18F-FDG PET versus iliac biopsy in the initial evaluation of bone marrow infiltration in the case of Hodgkin's disease: a meta-analysis. Nucl Med Commun 2013;34(1):25–31.
35. Devenney-Cakir B, Subramaniam RM, Reddy SM, et al. Cystic and cystic-appearing lesions of the mandible: review. Am J Roentgenol 2011;196(6):WS66–77.
36. Harada H, Takinami S, Makino S. Three-phase bone scintigraphy and viability of vascularized bone grafts for mandibular reconstruction. Int J Oral Maxillofac Surg 2000;29(4):280–4.

37. Moskowitz GW, Lukash F. Evaluation of bone graft viability. Semin Nucl Med 1988; 18(3):246–54.
38. Furr MC, Cannady S, Nance R, et al. The use of nuclear bone scanning after fibula free tissue transfer. Laryngoscope 2013;123(12):2980–5.
39. Lauer I, Czech N, Zieron J, et al. Assessment of the viability of microvascularized bone grafts after mandibular reconstruction by means of bone SPECT and semi-quantitative analysis. Eur J Nucl Med 2000;27(10):1552–6.
40. Berding G, Burchert W, van den Hoff J, et al. Evaluation of the incorporation of bone grafts used in maxillofacial surgery with [18F]fluoride ion and dynamic positron emission tomography. Eur J Nucl Med 1995;22(10):1133–40.
41. Ruggiero SL, Dodson TB, Fantasia J, et al. American association of oral and maxillofacial surgeons position paper on medication-related osteonecrosis of the jaw: 2014 update. J Oral Maxillofac Surg 2014;72(10):1938–56.
42. de Castro LA, de Castro JG, de Alcantara JS, et al. Why physicians should look at the mouths of their patients. J Clin Med Res 2016;8(12):841–3.
43. Khan AA, Morrison A, Hanley DA, et al. Diagnosis and management of osteonecrosis of the jaw: a systematic review and international consensus. J Bone Miner Res 2015;30(1):3–23.
44. Guggenberger R, Fischer DR, Metzler P, et al. Bisphosphonate-induced osteonecrosis of the jaw: comparison of disease extent on contrast-enhanced MR imaging, [18F] fluoride PET/CT, and conebeam CT imaging. AJNR Am J Neuroradiol 2013;34(6):1242–7.
45. Wilde F, Steinhoff K, Frerich B, et al. Positron-emission tomography imaging in the diagnosis of bisphosphonate-related osteonecrosis of the jaw. Oral Surg Oral Med Oral Pathol Oral Radiol Endod 2009;107(3):412–9.
46. Dammacco F, Rubini G, Ferrari C, et al. ^{18}F-FDG PET/CT: a review of diagnostic and prognostic features in multiple myeloma and related disorders. Clin Exp Med 2015;15(1):1–18.
47. Wilde F, Steinhoff K, Frerick B, et al. Positron-emission tomography imaging in the diagnosis of bisphosphonate-related osteonecrosis of the jaw. Oral and maxillofacial radiology 2009;107(3):412–9.

Moving?

Make sure your subscription moves with you!

To notify us of your new address, find your **Clinics Account Number** (located on your mailing label above your name), and contact customer service at:

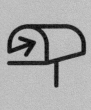

Email: journalscustomerservice-usa@elsevier.com

800-654-2452 (subscribers in the U.S. & Canada)
314-447-8871 (subscribers outside of the U.S. & Canada)

Fax number: 314-447-8029

Elsevier Health Sciences Division
Subscription Customer Service
3251 Riverport Lane
Maryland Heights, MO 63043

*To ensure uninterrupted delivery of your subscription, please notify us at least 4 weeks in advance of move.

ELSEVIER